Forensic gynaecology

Towards better care for the female victim of sexual assault

Forensic gynaecology

Towards better care for the female victim of sexual assault

Edited by Maureen Dalton

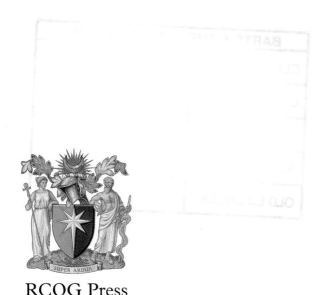

RCOG Press

Published by the **RCOG Press** at the Royal College of Obstetricians and Gynaecologists, 27 Sussex Place, Regent's Park, London NW1 4RG

www.rcog.org.uk

Registered charity no. 213280

First published 2004

ISBN 1 900364 84 0

RCOG Press Editor: Jane Moody
Design: Karl Harrington, FiSH Books
Printed by Latimer Trend & Co. Ltd., Estover Road, Plymouth PL6 7PL

Contents

Contributors

Helen Cameron FRCOG
Consultant Obstetrician and Gynaecologist, Sunderland Royal Hospital, Kayll Road, Sunderland SR4 7TP, UK.

Judith Common
Superintendent, Corporate Services, Northumbria Police, Performance Review and Inspectorate Headquarters, Ponteland, Newcastle upon Tyne NE20 0BL, UK.

Maureen Dalton MRCS LRCP FRCOG
Consultant Obstetrician and Gynaecologist, Royal Devon & Exeter Hospital (Heavitree), Gladstone Road, Exeter EX1 2AD, UK.

Camille de San Lazaro OBE
Consultant Paediatrician and Senior Lecturer in Paediatric Forensic Medicine, The Lindisfarne Centre, Royal Victoria Infirmary, Queen Victoria Road, Newcastle upon Tyne NE1 4LP, UK.

Ruby Hamid
Barrister, 18 Red Lion Court, London EC4A 3EB, UK.

Joseph K Johnson MD DGO MRCOG
Specialist Registrar, Hull Maternity Hospital, Hedon Road, Hull HU9 5LX, UK.

Gillian Jones
Barrister, 18 Red Lion Court, London EC4A 3EB, UK.

Stephen Lindow FCOG(SA) FRCOG
Senior Lecturer in Perinatology, Hull Maternity Hospital, Hedon Road, Hull HU9 5LX, UK.

Kate Mulley
Policy Manager, Victim Support National Office, Cranmer House, 39 Brixton Road, London SW9 6DZ

Mary Newton
Senior Forensic Scientist, Metropolitan Police, London Forensic Science
Laboratory, 109 Lambeth Road, London SE1 7LP, UK.

Mary Pillai MD DCH MRCP(UK) MRCPCH FRCOG
Consultant Obstetrician and Gynaecologist and Forensic Medical
Examiner, St Paul's Wing, Cheltenham General Hospital, Sandford Road,
Cheltenham GL53 7AN, UK.

Helen Reeves DBE
Chief Executive, Victim Support, National Office, Cranmer House,
39 Brixton Road, London SW9 6OZ, UK.

Raine E I Roberts MBE
Cinical Director (retired), Sexual Assault Referral Centre, St Mary's
Hospital, Whitworth Park, Manchester M13 0JH, UK.

Deborah Rogers DCH DRCOG MRCGP DFFP MMJ
Principal Forensic Medical Examiner for Thames Valley Police and
Medical Director Swindon Sanctuary Sexual Assault Referral Centre,
Taw Hill Medical Practice, Queen Elizabeth Drive, Swindon, Wiltshire
SN25 1WL, UK.

Peter Rook QC
Barrister and Head of Chambers, 18 Red Lion Court, London EC4A
3EB, UK.

Lindsey Stevens MA FRCP FFAEM FRSA
Honorary Senior Lecturer, St George's Hospital Medical School, and
Director, Accident and Emergency Services, Epsom and St Helier
University NHS Trust, Wrythe Lane, Carshalton, Surrey SM5 1AA, UK.

Hazel Walter DRCOG DFFP MRCGP DMJ(Clinical)
Forensic Physician, West Mercia Constabulary Headquarters, Hindlip
Hall, Hindlip, PO Box 55, Worcester WR3 8SP, UK.

Jan Welch FRCP
Consultant in Genitourinary Medicine, Clinical Director of the Haven –
Camberwell, King's College Hospital, Denmark Hill, London SE5 9RS,
UK.

Michael Wilks
Chairman, Medical Ethics Committee, British Medical Association, BMA
House, Tavistock Square, London WC1H 9JP, UK.

Foreword

Rape is a topic that is not covered in the undergraduate curriculum and it is only just starting to enter the postgraduate curriculum. While male rape is a serious and under-reported crime, this book covers forensic gynaecology specifically and so male sexual assault is not discussed. This is not meant to deny the issue of male rape; indeed, much of the book is pertinent to the forensic examination of the male complainant.

According to the British Crime Survey 2002,[1] one in 20 women is the victim of a sexual assault. In the year 2000, this equated to approximately 61 000 women. The majority of sexual assaults are not reported to the police and domestic or spousal rape is even less commonly reported. We do know, however, that women who are the victims of sexual assault are more likely to use the health service so we, as medical practitioners, will see them in our day-to-day practice. Optimising the care of the victim of sexual assault is bound to alleviate some of the subsequent health problems that she may experience. As a gynaecologist, I have a duty to try to provide the best health care to women. This includes ensuring that the medical needs of the victim of rape are recognised in conjunction with providing support for complainants at all stages of the process of clinical and forensic management.

If we are to improve our response to rape cases we need to improve the levels of communication between the forensic medical examiner, the general practitioner, counsellors, police, Crown Prosecution Service and, not least, the complainant herself. It is with this in mind that the Royal College of Obstetricians and Gynaecologists arranged to hold study days on the topic of forensic gynaecology.

To reflect the needs of all potential forensic examiners, this book has a multidisciplinary basis and has been designed on two levels. To assist the doctor with little or no knowledge on the subject, the first part of each chapter is devoted to an explanation of the relevant facts. Each topic covered has areas of debate and some of the controversies are explored in the second part of each chapter, subtitled 'the dilemmas', where we have endeavoured to provide a stimulus for discussion. The aim of this book is to be of interest to both the experts and the newcomer to the subject.

The Government has just reformed the laws relating to sexual offences and Peter Rook, Gillian Jones and Ruby Hamid discuss these changes in Chapter 1. It has been a Herculean task for them to rewrite the chapter so quickly. The act was only passed at the end of November 2003.

There is a continuum involving rape which also includes child sex abuse and domestic violence and so these equally unacceptable forms of violence against women are also discussed. The main focus is on the management of the woman who discloses that she has been raped. The term **complainant** has been used to emphasise that it is the role of the court and not the doctor to decide if she is a **victim** of rape.

One of the reasons why this is such a challenging area in which to work is the dual role of the examiner to look after the health needs of the complainant at the same time as collecting and often interpreting forensic evidence. We are constantly looking for ways of improving evidence gathering. The forensic examiner is ever mindful of the welfare of the complainant and yet must fulfil another dual role of remaining impartial, although empathetic, towards to the woman.

Finally, I must thank the many people who have helped in this project and especially the chapter contributors. My consultant colleague, Helen Cameron, has suffered not only because, during the writing phase, she too shared in the Northumbria Police Forensic Medical Examiner rota but also in that her office was next to mine, where she was all too readily accessible to mull over editorial detail. This book would not exist but for the hard work put in by Jane Moody, Sophie Leighton and Michael Ewins at the RCOG. Thanks to email, I could happily work at antisocial hours and they could reply at civilised times.

Maureen Dalton
April 2004

Reference

1.   British Crime Survey 2002. [www.homeoffice.gov.uk/rds/bcs1.html].

SECTION ONE
Rape: the facts and the dilemmas

Chapter 1

The law of rape

Peter Rook, Gillian Jones and Ruby Hamid

Introduction

Rape is often regarded as the most serious sexual offence although there may
be severe degradation of the victim during an indecent assault. In the 1990s,
the law of rape underwent significant change in order to go some way towards
addressing the criticisms of the way sexual offences are defined in England and
Wales. The effect of those changes was firstly to widen the category of persons
who may be raped and secondly to widen the definition of what constitutes
rape. In the 1992 case of R v R,[1] the exception to the law of rape whereby a
man could not be found guilty of raping his wife was finally and completely
abrogated. The Criminal Justice and Public Order Act 1994 altered the basis
of the offence by enacting that rape included penetration of the anus, with the
result that a man as well as a woman may be the victim of rape.

In 1999, the Government embarked upon a wholesale review of the law in
relation to sexual offences. This has resulted in the Sexual Offences Act 2003.
Much of the law dated from 19th-century laws that codified the common law
at the time and reflected the social attitudes and roles of men and women at
that time. This piece of legislation consolidates the law in relation to sexual
offences under one umbrella. The aim of the new legislation is to modernise
the law relating to sexual offences by bringing the language and terminology
into the 21st century. Particular emphasis is also placed on the protection of
children from sexual crime. The changes, as they come into force, will
significantly alter the law as it currently stands. The new law, as far as it relates
to rape, is set out under each heading, so the old and new positions can be
contrasted as far as is possible within the scope of this work.

The definition of rape

Old law (all offences committed before 1 May 2004)

Until 1976, there was no statutory definition of rape. Rape was defined at
common law as unlawful sexual intercourse with a woman without her

consent, by force, fear or fraud.[2] This definition was potentially misleading. In 1975, widespread concern was expressed by the public, the media and in Parliament in response to the decision of the House of Lords in DPP v Morgan and Others.[3] This led the Home Secretary to appoint a committee under the chairmanship of Mrs Justice Heilbron to give urgent consideration to the law of rape. The Committee recommended that the time had come for a statutory definition of rape: "this would provide the opportunity to clarify the existing law and in particular to bring out the importance of recklessness as a mental element in the crime. Such a definition would also emphasise that a lack of consent (and not violence) is the crux of the matter".[4]

Section 1(1) of the Sexual Offences (Amendment) Act 1976 incorporated the Committee's recommendation into the Sexual Offences Act 1956, providing a statutory definition of rape. Section 1(1) has since been repealed by section 142 of the Criminal Justice and Public Order Act 1994, which substituted a new section 1 into the Sexual Offences Act 1956. The effect of the change is to extend the definition of rape to encompass anal intercourse with a woman or a man. A further effect was to remove the word 'unlawful' from the definition, thereby confirming that rape within a marriage is an offence. The statutory definition of rape for offences committed before 1 May 2004 is given in Box 1.1.[5]

Box 1.1 Statutory definition of rape: old law

Sexual Offences Act 1956, section 1

Rape of woman or man

1 It is an offence for a man to rape a woman or another man.

2 A man commits rape if:
 (a) he has sexual intercourse with a person (whether vaginal or anal) who, at the time of the intercourse, does not consent to it; and
 (b) at the time, he knows that the person does not consent to the intercourse or is reckless as to whether that person consents to it.

3 A man also commits rape if he induces a married woman to have sexual intercourse with him by impersonating her husband.

4 Subsection (2) applies for the purposes of any enactment.

Sexual Offences (Amendment) Act 1976, section 1

1 [Repealed by Criminal Justice and Public Order Act 1994, section 168(3) and Schedule 11.]

2 It is hereby declared that, if at a trial for a rape offence, the jury has to consider whether a man believed that a woman or man was consenting to sexual intercourse, the presence or absence of reasonable grounds for such a belief is a matter to which the jury is to have regard, in conjunction with any other relevant matters, in considering whether he so believed.[6]

New law (offences committed after 1 May 2004)

The new statutory framework is set out in Part 1 of the Sexual Offences Act 2003. In particular, sections 1–9 deal with rape and associated offences. Of importance, is the new definition of rape at section 1 (Box 1.2).

Box 1.2 Statutory definition of rape: new law

Sexual Offences Act 2003, Section 1

1   A person (A) commits an offence if:
   (a) he intentionally penetrates the vagina, anus or mouth of another person (B) with his penis
   (b) B does not consent to the penetration, and
   (c) A does not reasonably believe that B consents.

2   Whether a belief is reasonable is to be determined having regard to all the circumstances, including any steps A has taken to ascertain whether B consents.

This brings forced oral intercourse into the definition of rape; the basis for that being that "forced oral sex is as horrible, as demeaning and as traumatising as other forms of forced penile penetration".[6] Evidentially securing sufficiently clear forensic evidence as to forced oral sexual intercourse may well be very difficult.

There is still a requirement on the prosecution to establish lack of consent on the part of the complainant as to the alleged penetration. The defence of a genuinely held but unreasonable belief in consent has been abolished. The focus will now be on whether the prosecution can establish the absence of a reasonable belief by the defendant that the complainant was consenting. Consent will be dealt with more fully later in the chapter.

In keeping with the objectives of the new legislation, namely to reduce sexual crime that relates to children, a new offence is set out at section 5 of the Sexual Offences Act 2003: rape of a child under 13 (Box 1.3). This is an offence of strict liability once intentional penetration with the penis is established. In contrast to the old law, if the complainant is under 13 years of age, they are deemed incapable of consent and therefore the defendant would be guilty even if the child were a willing party to the act. There are defences of mistaken belief as to consent, or as to the age of the child, even if it is reasonable in the circumstances. An extreme example of the implications of the change in law would be a situation where a 12-year-old girl performs fellatio on her 13-year-old boyfriend. Both are consenting parties but their relationship breaks down and she tells her parents what they have done. The parents wish to press charges and the child, because of familial pressure, agrees. Under the Act, the young boy would be a rapist.

Much will depend upon the discretion of the prosecuting authorities as to which cases warrant prosecution.

Box 1.3 Statutory definition of rape of a child under 13 years

Sexual Offences Act 2003, Section 5

1 A person commits an offence if:
   (a) he intentionally penetrates the vagina, anus or mouth of another person with his penis, and
   (b) the other person is under 13 years.

Mode of trial and punishment

The old law

Both rape and attempted rape are triable only on indictment, which means that they can only be tried in the Crown Court, except for certain cases involving very young defendants where there is provision for summary trial.[7] Rape and attempted rape are class 2 offences,[8] triable only by a High Court judge, except under special circumstances. The maximum penalty on a charge of rape or attempted rape is life imprisonment.[9]

The new law

The penalties for rape, including the new offence of rape of a child under 13 years, remain the same under the new Act. New offences of assault by penetration and sexual assault will replace indecent assault. Assault by penetration is the most serious, with a maximum sentence of life imprisonment. Sexual assault will be triable either in the Magistrates Court or the Crown Court , with a maximum penalty of ten years when tried in the Crown Court. There are parallel offences for children under 13 years; namely, assault by penetration of a child under 13 years (consent is not an element) and sexual assault on a child under 13 years: again, to which consent is not an issue. The maximum penalty is 14 years' imprisonment.

Ingredients of the offence

Parties to the offence

Old law

Only a man[10] can commit the offence of rape as a principal but a woman may be convicted of aiding and abetting a man to commit rape. Indeed, a woman who encourages or assists a man to have sexual intercourse with another woman, knowing that the other woman does not consent, may be found guilty of aiding and abetting rape, notwithstanding that the man is acquitted of rape on the ground that he mistakenly believed that the woman was consenting.

The presumption in law that a boy under the age of 14 years is incapable of vaginal or anal intercourse was abolished by section 1 of the Sexual Offences Act 1993. The prosecution still has to prove, where the defendant is under the age of 14 years, that he knew that what he was doing was wrong.

New law

Under the Sexual Offences Act 2003, again, only a man can commit the offence of rape as a principle.

The physical act

Old law: sexual intercourse, vaginal or anal

To prove that sexual intercourse took place, the prosecution must prove that the defendant's penis penetrated the victim's vagina or anus. The slightest penetration is sufficient and, in respect of the hymen, it is not necessary to show that it was ruptured. In Lines, the victim's hymen had not been ruptured but a venereal sore had developed upon it. Parke J. ruled that if any part of the virile member of the defendant was within the labia of the pudendum of the victim, no matter how little, this would be sufficient.[11] Whether the defendant ejaculated during the period of penetration is irrelevant. Thus, there is no requirement to prove completion of the intercourse by the 'emission of seed'.[12]

Although sexual intercourse is deemed complete upon penetration, it is a continuing act, which continues as long as penetration is maintained and ends only with withdrawal. It follows that, if a defendant becomes aware that the woman is not consenting after penetration but before withdrawal and then continues the act of intercourse, he commits the act of rape (the other elements being present).[13]

New law: penetration of vagina, anus or mouth

As with the previous definition, the offence is complete on penetration no matter how slight. This now includes any penetration of the mouth. There need not be ejaculation. Section 79(2) of the Act, re-establishes the principle that intercourse is a continuing act. Therefore, it follows that the offence is committed in circumstances where the defendant penetrates the victim and subsequently becomes aware that he or she is not consenting but continues nevertheless. Section 79(9) makes it clear that vagina includes vulva, while section 79(3) states that references to a part of the body include references to a part surgically constructed, in particular through gender reassignment surgery.

Absence of consent

Old law

The prosecution must prove that, at the time of the sexual intercourse, the woman did not consent to it and that the defendant either knew that the victim was not consenting or that he was reckless as to whether she or he was consenting.[14] This is so, whatever the victim's age: there is no statutory age limit below which a child is incapable of consent. In reality, with a very young complainant, the prosecution will not need to prove much more than her age.[15] Sexual intercourse and the absence of consent are the vital physical elements of the offence. Evidence of nonconsensual sexual intercourse covers a wide variety of factual circumstances: a straight refusal by the victim which is communicated to the defendant, use of force (although often present in rape, it is not an essential ingredient), where the victim was deceived as to the identity of the defendant,[16] where the victim was unaware as to what was happening and/or was incapable of giving consent due to drink,[17] drugs, sleep,[18] age[19] or mental handicap.[20]

A jury should be directed by the trial judge that the word 'consent' carries its ordinary meaning. In some circumstances the judge may need to give a direction on which forms of pressure might vitiate consent where there has been no violence or threat of violence. In Olugboja,[21] the Court recognised that consent is not an entirely straightforward concept for a jury, covering as it does a wide spectrum of states of mind, ranging from actual desire on the one hand to reluctant acquiescence on the other. The court stated that, in that situation, the issue of consent should not be left to the jury without some further direction.[22] Where a distinction between real consent and mere submission is to be drawn, it is a matter for the jury to decide, "applying their combined good sense, experience and knowledge of human nature and modern behaviour to all the relevant facts of the case". In a later case of MacAllister,[23] an indecent assault, the jury had sent a note asking for assistance about the difference between submission and consent. Counsel for the appellant persuaded the trial judge not to give a dictionary definition to the jury. On appeal, Brooke L.J. said that the trial judge could not have been faulted if he had given the jury the proposed dictionary definitions: "to submit ... to give way, resign oneself, yield, cease or abstain from resistance" contrasted with the words "to consent ... to express willingness, give permission, agree". He also stated that the jury would not necessarily have been helped by a reference to reluctant acquiescence.[23]

Other evidence that is capable of assisting a jury to determine the issue of consent includes the lack of sexual experience of a complainant and her attitudes and religious beliefs that intercourse before marriage was wrong.[24]

Consent obtained by deception

Under the 1956 Act, two types of deception vitiated consent: deception as to the nature of the sexual act and deception as to the identity of the perpetrator.

An example of the first type is where the victim is induced to consent because she is told that intercourse is a form of medical treatment. It would appear that if the complainant makes a fundamental mistake as to the nature of the act, there is no consent, whether or not the mistake is obtained by deception. An example of the second type is where a man impersonates the complainant's husband (section 1(2) of the Sexual Offences Act 1956). The case of Elbekkay expanded the offence to cover impersonation of the complainant's welcome sexual partner, as well as her husband.

Mental capacity of the complainant

The mental capacity of the complainant is important when considering the issue of consent. Where a complainant is mentally ill or subnormal, he or she may not be capable of consenting to sexual intercourse. Under the old law, there were no clear principles governing whether a person had capacity to consent to sexual acts: it was a question of fact for the jury to determine in accordance with their interpretation of the ordinary meaning of the word 'consent'. Clearly, a complainant's capacity to consent depends upon the degree to which their understanding is impaired. A useful test of capacity was formulated in the Australian case of Morgan.[25] Under this test, it must be proved that a complainant is lacking sufficient knowledge or understanding to comprehend, a) that what is proposed to be done is the physical act of penetration of her body by the male organ, or if that is not proved, b) that the act of penetration proposed is one of sexual connection, as distinct from an act of a totally different nature. If, on the application of this test, a woman is found to be incapable of consenting, then a man having intercourse with her commits rape if he knows that she does not consent or is reckless as to whether or not she consents.

There was no special provision to cover a situation where the complainant's behaviour was influenced by drink or drugs at the time of intercourse but this has been addressed by the Court of Appeal and certain principles have been established. Where a victim's will is weakened without the use of threats or fraud, a seducer does not commit rape if the victim consents knowing what is happening. The crucial question is not why the victim took the drink or drugs but whether she understood the situation and was in a position to decide whether to consent or resist.[26] If a jury finds that a complainant was in such a state of inebriation that she was not able to exercise a judgement on the question of consent, the prosecution would have succeeded in establishing absence of consent.[27]

If the complainant is asleep at the time of intercourse she is incapable of consenting.[28] In this situation, rape can be established on the basis that absence of consent is sufficient; it is not necessary for the complainant to positively dissent. A problem arises where the parties have slept regularly together and had consensual intercourse in the past, although there may not be specific consent by the complainant on the occasion alleged, the mental element for rape on the part of the man may not be present.[29]

The issue of consent and rape where the parties are in a long-term relationship was addressed by the Court of Appeal in R v Mohammed Zafar,[30] a case where the defendant and complainant had a long-standing relationship and had lived together for a long time. The court approved the trial judge's summing-up to the jury as an admirable exposition of the law. The trial judge, J Pill, had said the fact that the parties were in a long-standing relationship was evidence that should be taken into consideration and, although a woman may not particularly want intercourse on a particular occasion, in practice she will consent reluctantly because it is her partner who is asking for it. He continued, "however, a woman is entitled to say 'no' and to refuse consent even to her husband or long-term partner ... it is for you to decide whether the absence of consent is proved in this case".

Consent under the 2003 Act

The new definition of consent can be found at section 74 of the Sexual Offences Act 2003. It remains a requirement for the prosecution to prove that the complainant did not consent. Consent under the Act is now set out as follows: "a person consents if he agrees by choice and has the freedom and capacity to make that choice".

Capacity to consent

'Capacity' is not defined in the 2003 Act. However, the Act creates distinct offences which cover the main areas where the capacity of the complainant to consent tends to arise. For instance, section 5 of the Act makes penile penetration of a child below 13 years of age an offence of rape, irrespective of whether the child consented. The Act creates a series of offences to protect those with mental disorders (as defined by section 1 of the Mental Health Act 1965). Furthermore, under section 30 of the Act, penetrative sex with a person unable to refuse by reason of a mental disorder becomes an offence carrying a maximum sentence of life imprisonment.

The mental element

Old law

As well as the physical elements (intercourse and absence of consent), the defendant's state of mind is vital to the offence. He can only be convicted under the current law if he knew that the victim did not consent or was reckless about whether or not the victim did consent. As stated in section 1(2) of the Sexual Offences (Amendment) Act 1976,[31] if the jury has to consider whether the defendant believed the victim to be consenting, it must consider the presence or absence of reasonable grounds for that belief along with any other relevant matters in its decision-making process. 'Other relevant matters' may include the defendant's conduct up to the time of the alleged rape.[32] Section 1(2) should be read alongside the case of Morgan,[33] which said that if a defendant is under a mistaken belief that the victim consented he cannot be guilty of rape, even if he had no reasonable grounds for such a belief.

Whenever there is scope on the facts for the jury to find that the defendant had a genuine but mistaken belief that the complainant was consenting, the judge should direct the jury that if the defendant may have had such a belief, they should acquit.[34] There is no general requirement that the jury must be directed in this way – it will depend on the evidence.[35] The burden to disprove a defence of 'mistaken belief' in consent rests with the prosecution; this jury direction was suggested by the Court of Appeal in Gardiner: "Has the Crown eliminated the possibility of a genuine though mistaken belief?".[36]

Recklessness

The decade following Morgan[37] and the 1976 Amendment Act saw some important decisions as to the meaning of recklessness in the Criminal Law. In Satnam and Kewal,[37] the Court of Appeal cited with approval the practical definition of LJ Lawton in Kimber:[38] if the jury was sure that the defendant had been indifferent to the feelings and wishes of the victim, aptly described as "couldn't care less" then, in law, that was "reckless". This approach was further endorsed by the Court of Appeal in the case of Taylor,[39] which simplified the definition of reckless rape to this: "in rape the defendant is reckless if he does not believe that the woman is consenting and could not care less whether she is consenting or not but presses on regardless".

Self-induced intoxication by the defendant cannot be used as the basis for the denial of the mental element of rape. It was held in Fotheringham[40] that no mistake, whether as to consent or any other matter, arising from self-induced intoxication can be a defence to rape. On the facts of that case, the defendant's defence to raping the babysitter was that he was so drunk that he mistakenly believed he was having intercourse with his wife. The Court of Appeal upheld the trial judge's direction that the jury had to consider whether the grounds for the defendant's belief would have seemed reasonable to a sober man.

For a man to be convicted of conspiracy to rape, recklessness as to whether the victim consents is not sufficient.[41] He must have knowledge of all the physical elements of the offence, including the absence of consent. Accordingly, for conspiracy to rape to be established, there must be an agreement with at least one other to have intercourse with a victim, knowing that he or she will not consent. If the agreement is to have intercourse with a victim not knowing whether there will be consent or not, there is no conspiracy to rape. However, as soon as acts are performed that are more than merely preparatory, an attempted rape is committed.

The new Act abolishes the defence that the defendant had a genuine but unreasonably held belief that the complainant was consenting. In those circumstances, the defendant would no longer be entitled to an acquittal. The issue is, therefore, whether the defendant held an honest and 'reasonable' belief that the victim was consenting, having regard to all the circumstances, including any steps the defendant has taken at the time to ascertain whether the complainant was consenting. It is not yet clear to what extent a jury will be entitled to take into account the personal characteristics of the defendant when considering whether his belief was reasonable. There seems little doubt that such characteristics as youth and learning disability can be considered by the jury.

The prosecution can establish lack of consent in three ways:

- it was not 'reasonable' to hold that belief in all the circumstances
  This question will be a matter for the jury to determine, looking at both the individuals concerned and the surrounding circumstances.

- to rely on one of the 'evidential' presumptions set out in section 75:
  (i)   that any person used and/or threatened violence against the complainant at the time of the act or immediately before the first sexual activity began
  (ii)   that any person caused the complainant to fear at the time of the act or immediately before the first sexual act that violence was being used or would be used immediately against another person
  (iii) that the complainant was, and the defendant was not, unlawfully detained at the time
  (iv)   that the complainant was asleep or otherwise unconscious at the time
  (v)   that the complainant's physical disability renders her unable to communicate to the defendant whether she consents
  (vi)   that any person had administered to or caused to be taken by the complainant, without the complainant's consent, a substance which, having regard to when it was administered or taken, was capable of causing or enabling the complainant to be stupefied or overpowered at the time of the relevant act.

The evidential presumption operates in the following way. If the prosecution have proved that the defendant committed the act of intentional penetration and it is proved that any one of the circumstances listed above existed, and the defendant knew it existed, the complainant is presumed not to have consented and for the defendant not to have had a reasonable belief in her consent. This presumption can be rebutted if the judge is satisfied, at the close of all the evidence, that sufficient evidence has been adduced to raise an issue as to consent or belief in consent. The prosecution must then prove absense of consent and unreasonable belief beyond reasonable doubt.

Only one of the circumstances must be proved before the presumption bites. The defendant has to know that the circumstance exists but there is no requirement that the circumstance actually caused the victim's lack of consent. It is, in effect, simply presumed. The threat of or use of violence does not necessarily have to come from the defendant himself. The threat must be immediate rather than something that may happen in the future.

■ to rely on one of the "conclusive" presumptions set out in section 76:

It shall be conclusively presumed that the victim did not consent if the defendant:
(a) intentionally deceived the victim as to the nature or purpose of the relevant act, or
(b) intentionally induced the victim to consent to the relevant act by impersonating a person known personally to the victim.

These circumstances involve deception; if one of them (along with the act of penetration) is proved by the prosecution, it is to be conclusively presumed that the complainant did not consent and that the defendant did not believe the complainant consented. There is no room for the defendant to adduce evidence to the contrary. The Act does not directly address the issue of deception about personal attributes (such as being a doctor, priest or policeman) but it does expand the categories of impersonation beyond the current law of husband or regular sexual partner.

The new definition of consent is an improvement, in that it is underpinned by the concept of free agreement, which will help to emphasise to juries that any agreement must be genuine and obtained without duress. However, the parameters of consent are still unclear. For instance, if a person is incapable of consenting through drink or the influence of drugs, they cannot consent, but what degree of incapacity is required? How is 'freedom' to be defined? Does it go beyond freedom from physical pressure to encompass such issues as cultural, economic or religious pressures? These are all questions for the future.

Evidential issues

Recent complaint

Evidence that a complainant made a consistent complaint to another person, shortly after the alleged offence, may be given in evidence at trial, as an exception to the rule against hearsay. The mere complaint is not evidence of the facts complained of and its admissibility depends upon proof of the facts by sworn testimony. In order to be admissible, the complaint must be made on the first reasonable opportunity after the offence and be a spontaneous statement, in the sense that it is an unassisted and unvarnished story of what happened. If admitted by the court, such a complaint can be relied on as being consistent with the sworn evidence of the complainant. However, it does not constitute corroboration, as it does not come from an independent source. The jury must, in all cases, be directed as to the limited weight to be attached to such evidence. The rule has been criticised on the basis that there may be powerful reasons why a complaint has not been made at the first opportunity. Under provisions in the Criminal Justice Act, all complaints will be admissible as evidence of the facts complained of.

Restrictions on evidence in trials of rape offences

Cross-examination of the complainant as to her previous sexual history

In December 1975, the Heilbron Committee recommended that some curtailment of unnecessary cross-examination of the complainant as to her sexual history was one of the most urgent and important reforms required. As a result, Parliament enacted section 2 of the Sexual Offences (Amendment) Act 1976, which provided that, where a defendant pleads not guilty to rape, "no evidence and no question in cross-examination shall be adduced at the trial . . . about any sexual experience of a complainant with a person other than that defendant. The judge shall not give leave except on an application made to him in the absence of the jury . . . and on such an application the judge shall give leave . . . if he is satisfied it would be unfair to that defendant to refuse to allow the evidence to be adduced or the question to be asked". Thus, no question may be asked about, nor evidence adduced of the complainant's previous sexual history with anyone other than the defendant, without leave of the judge, and leave will only be granted if he is satisfied that it would be unfair to the defendant to refuse to do so.

Section 2 was criticised heavily on the basis that judges were allowing too many applications. This led to the repeal of section 2, which has now been replaced by sections 41–43 of the Youth Justice and Criminal Evidence Act 1999 [YJCEA]. These provisions place a general prohibition on the admissibility of previous sexual history evidence unless the court gives leave. Section 41(1) YJCEA provides that: "If at trial a person is charged with a sexual offence, then, except with the leave of the Court: (a) no evidence may be adduced, and (b) no questions may be asked in cross-examination, by or on behalf of any accused at the trial, about any sexual behaviour of the complainant".

Significantly, section 41(1) does not include the words, 'with a person other than the defendant'. There is no longer a presumption that previous sexual experience/behaviour with the defendant is relevant to consent. Leave must be sought and the appropriate tests applied even if the complainant and defendant are married or have a continuing sexual relationship.

Parliament made this change without any significant intellectual debate. The correct approach in respect of sexual behaviour with the defendant on other occasions has now been clarified by the House of Lords in the case of R v A (No 2) [2001]. The new test falls into two parts.

Part One

The court may not give leave unless it is satisfied that section 41(3) or 41(5) applies. Subsection 3 applies if the evidence or question relates to a relevant issue in the case and either:

(a)   Section 41(3) (a), where issue is not an issue of consent. This includes the defence of honest belief in consent under the old law and presumably will include reasonable belief in all the circumstances under the new law. Arguably, it also includes a case where there is evidence of bias on behalf of the complainant against the accused and/or a motive to fabricate the evidence. It must include an alternative explanation for the physical conditions on which the prosecution relies to establish that intercourse took place, such as injuries, disease or other medical evidence. It might include an explanation for a young complainant's knowledge of sexual practice.

(b)   Section 41(3)(b), where the issue is consent and the sexual behaviour of the complainant is 'at or about the same time as the event which is the subject matter of the charge against the accused'.

(c)   Section 41(3)(c), where the issue is consent and the sexual behaviour of the defendant is 'so similar . . . that the similarity cannot reasonably be explained as a coincidence'.

(d)   Section 41(4) allows evidence to rebut any evidence adduced by the prosecution about any sexual behaviour of the complainant which goes no further than necessary to enable that evidence to be rebutted or explained.

By virtue of Section 41(5), no evidence is to be regarded as relating to a relevant issue if it appears that the purpose (or main purpose) is to impugn the credibility of the complainant.

Part Two

Even if the proposed evidence or question falls within Section 41(a) to (c) or Section 41(5) and the hurdles of Section 41(4) (purpose not to impugn credibility) and subsection (6) (specific instances/not general reputation) have been surmounted, then it will be necessary for the Court to determine whether the second part of the section has been satisfied. The question is: 'Is the court satisfied that a refusal of leave might have the result of rendering unsafe a conclusion of the jury or (as the case may be) the court on any relevant issue in the case?'

On the face of the statute, the trial judge was given no residual discretion. However, following the House of Lords case in R v A [No 2][2002], if a judge finds that were he to exclude evidence, he would be depriving a defendant of a fair trial then the evidence should be admitted. It is now not permissible to argue that by virtue of a complainant's sexual experiences with other partners they are less credible or more likely to have consented (the correct approach to the twin myths). R v A (No 2) [2002] will not open the floodgates but it has unshackled judges from a legislative straightjacket that might otherwise have led them to exclude truly relevant evidence on an arbitrary basis (principally in the context of sexual relationships between defendants and complainants) and thereby to have endangered the fairness of the trial. In the case of sexual relationships with third parties, it will only be in rare cases that the trial judge will grant leave in relation to the issue of consent but the safety valve of Lord Steyn's test in R v A is now there should an exceptional factual situation arise.

Protection of the complainant as a witness

From the moment a complainant makes an allegation of rape, neither her name, nor her address, nor a still or moving picture of her may be published or broadcast if it is likely to lead to her being publicly identified.[42] Such prohibition lasts for the woman's lifetime. A person charged with rape can apply to a judge that the anonymity provision should not apply in relation to the complainant. Such an application is only likely to be granted in rare circumstances, such as if the publication of the complainant's name might induce likely witnesses to come forward and the defendant's defence at trial will be substantially prejudiced if the application were not granted. A debate is continuing as to whether there should be parity for sex case defendants, allowing them anonymity until conviction, given the social stigma attached to such alleged offending.

New provisions have come into effect to afford complainants in rape cases greater protection when they are giving evidence in court. This is to ensure best evidence is achieved. The Youth Justice and Criminal Evidence Act 1999 allows for special measures to be in place when a vulnerable witness, such as a complainant in a rape case, gives evidence about the alleged offence.[43] These measures include the use of screens to prevent the complainant from being seen by the defendant,[44] the giving of evidence by 'live link',[45] (a live television link enables the court to see and hear the evidence of a witness who is absent from the courtroom, the exclusion of particular people from the courtroom while the witness gives evidence,[46] the removal of wigs and gowns,[47] and the use of pre-recorded video evidence-in-chief[48] (not yet in force) and, in the future, cross-examination[49] and re-examination, although these sections are not yet in force. The provisions are designed to enable a witness to give their best-quality evidence and to encourage victims of rape not only to come forward and report the allegation but also to follow this through to trial.

The dilemma

The new law

The Sexual Offences Act 2003 represents the greatest overhaul of sexual offences legislation since Victorian times. Without doubt, a comprehensive review of the law relating to sexual offences was long overdue and the Government was correct to state that the law on sex offences, as it stood, was archaic, incoherent and discriminatory.[50] However, as with any substantial review of an area of law, a number of the amendments are controversial; in particular, the changes to the law of consent. An analysis of all the proposed changes falls outside the ambit of this chapter. It is hoped that changes to the substantive law combined with better care for the complainant will increase the very low conviction rate in rape cases.

References and notes

1. [1992] 1 A. C. 599.
2. 1 Hale 626; East P. C. 434.
3. [1976] A. C. 182.
4. VIII Summary of Recommendation, para 1(p. 36). The proposed definition was also designed to pre-empt the argument that the question of recklessness did not directly arise from the decision in Morgan in view of the question certified.
5. As printed by the Criminal Justice and Public Order Act 1994, s. 142.
6. Setting the Boundaries, para 2.8.5.
7. Hearn [1970] Crim. L. R. 175.
8. Velasquez [1996] 1 Cr. App. R. 155.
9. D. P. P. v Merrman [1973] A. C 584 overruling inter alia, Holley [1969] 53 Cr. App. R. 519.
10. By s. 46 of the 1956 Act the word 'man' in s. 1(1) of the 1956 Act includes 'boy'.
11. Hughes [1841] 9 C. & P. 752; Lines [1844] 1 C. & K. 393. In Lines the victim's hymen had not been ruptured, but a venereal sore had developed upon it. Parke J. ruled that if any part of the virile member of the defendant was within the labia of the pudendum of the victim, no matter how little, this would be sufficient to constitute penetration. See also Allen (Henry) [1839] 9 C. & P. 31; M'Rue [1838] 8 C. & P. 641.
12. S. 44 Sexual Offences Act 1956.
13. Kaitamaki v R [1985] A. C. 147.
14. Bradley [1910] 4 Cr. App. R. 225 where a conviction for rape was quashed after the commissioner at trial had failed to direct the jury that the onus of proof was upon the prosecution to show that the girl had not consented.
15. R v Harling, 26 Cr. App. R. 127, CCA.
16. R v Malone [1998] 2 Cr. App. R. 447 CA.
17. Camplin [1845] 1 Den. 89. This was the first instance of the wider interpretation of rape. R v Lang, 62 Cr. App. R. 50 CA.
18. Fletcher [1859] Bell 63; R v Mayers [1872] 12 Cox 311; R v Young [1878] 14 Cox 114.
19. R v Howard, 50 Cr. App. R. 56, CCA.
20. R v Barratt [1873] L. R. 2 C. C. R. 81; R v Pressy [1867] 10 Cox 635, CCR.
21. 1981] 3 ALL E. R. 443.
22. At p. 448 per Dunn LJ.
23. In McAllister [1997] Crim L. R. 233.
24. Amado-Taylor [2001] 8 Archbold News 1, CA; [2001] ECWA Crim. 1898.
25. 1970] V. R. 337 at 441.
26. Lang (1975) 62 Cr. App. R. 50.
27. Camplin (1845) 1 Den. 89.

28.   Mayers 91872) 12 Cox C. C. 311.
29.   Page (1846) 2 Cox C. C. 133.
30.   unreported case, June18, 1993, CA: No. 92/2762/W2; Pill J's direction commended by
      the Court of Appeal in McAllister, [1997] Crim. L. R. 233.
31.   see paragraph 2.2 ante.
32.   In McFall [1994] Crim. L. R. 226 the complainant said she had faked orgasms so well
      that the defendant might think she was consenting; the Court of Appeal said that 'other
      relevant matters' must include the fact that she had been abducted at gunpoint by the
      defendant that day.
33.   Morgan v D. P. P. [1976] A. C. 182.
34.   Satnam S, Kewal S. (1983) 78 Cr. App. R. 149.
35.   Adkins [2000] 2 All E. R. 185.
36.   1994] Crim. L. R. 455.
37.   see paragraph 11.1 ante.
38.   77 Cr. App. R. 225.
39.   Taylor (Robert) 80 Cr. App. R. 327.
40.   1989) 88 Cr. App. R. 206.
41.   s1(2) Criminal Law Act 1977.
42.   S. 158(2) Criminal Justice Act 1988, substituting s. 4(1) Sexual Offences
      (Amendment) Act 1976.
43.   S. 17 Youth Justice and Criminal Evidence Act 1999 (YJCEA) sets out special
      measures for witnesses eligible for assistance on the ground of fear or distress about
      testifying. S. 17(4) states that "where the complainant in respect of a sexual offence is a
      witness in proceedings relating to that offence. the witness is eligible for assistance in
      relation to those proceedings by virtue of this subsection".
44.   S. 23 YJCEA.
45.   s. 24 YJCEA.
46.   s. 25 YJCEA.
47.   s. 26 YJCEA.
48.   s. 27 YJCEA.
49.   s. 28 YJCEA.
50.   Protecting the Public. Home Office, November 2002 CM 5668.

Chapter 2
The police response
Judith Common

Introduction

Within this chapter an overview is given of the police response to victims of rape and serious sexual assault. It is widely acknowledged that the initial contact with the police and the subsequent contact between the victim and the continuing support offered are paramount in assisting in the overall recovery. It is also vital to help and support the individual through the investigative and subsequent judicial processes. In recent years there have also been significant developments in partnership working between the police and other supporting agencies, both statutory and non-statutory, which are able to offer continuing help and support. In addition, such agencies have been key in assisting the organisation to develop a deeper understanding of the complexities involved in the investigation and prosecution of such offences and the long-term impact upon the individual, the immediate family and the wider community.

This chapter is primarily concerned with the investigation and prosecution of rape and serious sexual assault on adult victims from a victim care perspective. It has been said that rape is the most serious survivable offence and it is acknowledged that such offences can cause significant emotional distress and psychological harm to the victim, which may take longer to overcome than any physical injuries.

The initial call

Rape is one of the most serious categories of crime and it is important that all steps are taken to encourage the victims of rape and serious sexual assault to report such offences. This objective is two-fold: it enables an investigation to begin, with a view to bringing the perpetrator to justice but, just as importantly, it enables the victim of such offences to access specialist help and support. With the significant advancement in forensic evidence, if an early report is made to the police service then arrangements can be made to obtain the necessary forensic samples. We should be and are proactive in encouraging victims of rape and sexual assault to come forward to report such instances. We are a much more victim-focused organisation and are committed to providing a service which takes cognisance of the individuals' needs, recognising diversity and cultural considerations.

Initial reports of rape are received in a similar manner to other categories of crime. The victim may make the initial call him- or herself to the emergency services or report in person to a police officer or at a police station. The call may also be made by a third party acting on behalf of the victim. What is highlighted in recent research is that it is important that the person who handles the first report treats the victim with sensitivity, is attentive and provides the victim with the time and space to make the initial report.[1] If the initial report is made at a police station, consideration should be given to the initial environment, which should afford privacy, be free of distractions and should minimise the risk of forensic contamination.

In light of developments in the provision of services to vulnerable victims and witnesses, many forces now have developed purpose-built facilities or co-located facilities within hospitals, social services premises or surgeries, which offer a safe, secure environment in which to carry out an initial report and to conduct a medical examination. While the provision of a bespoke facility may be costly, we need to be cognisant of the very real trauma that the victim may be suffering and in order to achieve the best possible evidence it is vital that both the attention to the wellbeing of the victim and the evidence-gathering process adhere to best practice principles. The significant developments and the provision of services to victims of rape and serious sexual assault need to be reinforced to encourage victims to come forward and report such cases. This is particularly relevant in the case of male victims and those from minority ethnic communities, who may perceive additional barriers to reporting such offences. A great deal of work has been carried out with the assistance of partner organisations and the provision of information leaflets in relevant languages but there is still a great deal more work to do in this area to reach and encourage all victims to report. The organisation is constantly looking at ways in which it can market the services provided through a variety of mediums.

The initial officer attending has a vital role to perform in order to provide the victim with the necessary support, preserve forensic evidence and provide assistance to the investigative team. It may well be that the initial report is to a member of support staff at a front counter or to a passing police patrol. There is a growing need for all officers and other personnel who have contact with the public to be trained to have an appreciation and awareness of victim care. This is now incorporated in many training programmes and, with the development of the National Competency Framework, victim and witness-related issues underpin much of the work in progress.

After the initial report is made, it is vital that a specialist officer who is trained in sexual offences investigative techniques is assigned to the victim at the earliest opportunity. The majority of forces have a cadre of officers who have the necessary skills, aptitude and training to undertake this work. In some forces, such officers are deployed as part of patrol teams and senior management ensures that a specialist officer is on duty to cover a cluster area at any given time, in other forces the officers are on an on-call rota and some forces operate an amalgam of the two. What is stressed is the importance of obtaining specialist provision at the earliest opportunity and victims should not have to wait excessive periods of time until a trained officer is available.

Training for sexual offences liaison officers

The training that specialist officers receive varies from force to force and there is growing pressure for national standards of competency to be developed. In one force (Northumbria) the initial training programme for sexual offences liaison officers is of three days duration. The officers are selected for the course by line management and, as such, all are volunteers who have completed a minimum of two years' service, have been trained in interview techniques and have attended a diversity development course. Upon the recommendations of senior management, the officers are selected for the training programme, which has the overall objective of preparing the officer to "understand the role of the sexual offences liaison officer, the need to support and guide the victim through the investigative process; liaise with the investigation team, access the services of REACH; have the required knowledge and skills to obtain an initial account of the rape from the victim".[2] REACH has two sexual assault referral centres that operate within the Northumbria Police Area. They are jointly funded by partners including health services, local authorities and police, and are operated by Northumbria Police with a multi-agency management team.

The course introduces officers to the forensic medical examination and the role of the forensic medical examiner, together with the principles of obtaining best evidence. Victim care issues, including rape trauma syndrome, is a key component of the course. The course outline is included as Appendix 2.1 to this chapter.

The medical examination

A medical examination will not be necessary in all cases of rape and serious sexual assault. For example, if the offence reported is an historic offence and the victim has only now felt strong enough to report the matter, a medical examination may not be necessary. In all cases, the decision to conduct a medical examination will be taken in collaboration with the sexual offences liaison officer, in consultation with the officer in charge of the case and the forensic medical examiner. The wishes of the victim will be paramount in reaching a decision.

In a recent rape or serious sexual assault, the importance of obtaining forensic samples, even if the victim is unsure whether they wish to support a police investigation, is vitally important. This can be accommodated and protocols have been built into the operating practices at some of the specialist centres, including St Mary's Hospital in Manchester and the REACH Centre in Northumbria, to enable samples to be taken while the victim is allowed the time and space to decide how they wish the matter to progress.

The arrangements for the medical examinations, together with the location, are critical to the wellbeing of the victim and to the obtaining of best evidence. The best possible service would be the provision of a specialist medical or multi-agency facility with continuing support and the choice of sex of the doctor carrying out the examination, who has a high level of expertise and training in this field. Historically, services and facilities have developed locally, based upon prevailing conditions, funding and logistics. Each force has developed services dependent upon local need and, as a result, there is a lack of uniformity in the services available to victims of rape and serious sexual assault. In April 2002, a joint inspection into the investigation and prosecution of cases involving allegations of rape was conducted by Her Majesty's Crown Prosecution Service Inspectorate and Her Majesty's Inspectorate of Constabulary (HMCPSI/HMIC).[1] They found that there were examples of good practice facilities at:

- St Mary's Hospital, Greater Manchester[3]
- The Juniper Centre, Leicester[4]
- The Haven–Camberwell, London[5]
- The REACH Centres, Northumbria.[6]

The advantages of such sexual assault referral centres are that victims can access a whole range of support from the outset, including counselling, health and welfare services.

In other instances, dedicated examination facilities, doctors' surgeries and joint examination facilities are used. It is important that any facility used takes into account the forensic and evidential needs as well as the care and professionalism that is necessary to the victim. This is of particular import-ance to minority ethnic victims and male victims who may have additional factors to overcome. As a result of the aforementioned report, forces were recommended to review existing facilities for victim examinations so that both victim care and integrity of evidence are maximised.

While we have concentrated on the physical environment and the continuing support at the time of the medical examination, the person who conducts the examination is critical when we consider that the forensic medical examiner has a key role to perform in the evidence gathering process. While it is important that the medical examiner has the requisite skills and training to carry out the examination it is also important that they are victim orientated and give support to the victim during the process. In the vast majority of forces, the forensic medical examiners are general practitioners who carry out the role in addition to their day-to-day responsibilities. Some forces use the police surgeon schemes and the examination of victims of rape and serious sexual assault is incorporated into those duties. In other areas, specialists are recruited who make up a cadre of individuals who, over time, build up a level of expertise that is recognised within the Criminal Justice System.

Within Northumbria Police, the women doctors scheme was launched in 1986. A significant number of female doctors, including consultant gynaecologists, paediatricians and experienced female general practitioners were recruited on a voluntary basis to provide a group of doctors willing to be placed on a call-out rota to conduct forensic medical examinations. Over a period of time, and with a continuing training and development programme, many doctors on the scheme have expert witness status. The scheme was extended to include male colleagues, in order to allow male victims of rape and serious sexual assault a gender-appropriate doctor to conduct the medical examination.

As a result of the formal make-up of the scheme, the training and mentoring programme undertaken, a considerable level of expertise has built up. There is the opportunity for peer review and a formalised meeting structure has developed, in which guest speakers from a variety of disciplines attend quarterly meetings. In addition, a structured training programme has been developed.

Another initiative worthy of note is the scheme under development at St Mary's Hospital, Manchester,[3] in which trained forensic nurses carry out the forensic medical examination. Once again, the key element is around the development of expertise and enhanced training for the role. The overall objective must always be to ensure that medical examination is carried out in a timely manner by a highly trained professional who has a sound appreciation and understanding of the forensic issues and, equally important, an awareness of victim care issues and the associated training surrounding rape.

The investigative process and the role of the sexual offences liaison officer

An important element of the liaison officer's role is as a conduit between the investigative team and the victim. As well as considering issues around victim care and continuing support, the officer is also a key player in the investigative process. The officer has a role to play in the obtaining of evidence, including an initial account of the offence and the compilation of an initial contact book. The officer is also required to keep the victim informed of the progress of the investigation in a way that takes into account the individual's needs.

In most instances, the sexual offences liaison officer is introduced to the victim at the earliest opportunity after the initial report, in order that they can immediately begin to build a productive working relationship. The

sexual offences liaison officer gives the victim timely and relevant information that allows the victim to make informed choices and remains with the
individual throughout the early hours of the complaint. The officer liaises
with the forensic medical examiner and, where a medical examination is
necessary, will accompany the victim during the medical examination. The
officer works as part of a team with the forensic medical examiner to ensure
that relevant samples are obtained and information recorded to ensure
continuity of evidence.

There is a high level of responsibility upon this officer and it is imperative
that officers have the correct aptitude, skills and training to carry out this
function. Because of the time constraints and the pressures often placed
upon these officers, it is vital that the overall workload is monitored and the
welfare needs of the officer are also addressed if we are to continue to
provide a professional service in this highly topical and emotive area of
police work.

Awareness is growing of rape trauma syndrome and the effects of post-
traumatic stress. It is in acknowledgement that the trauma of a recent attack
may inhibit full initial recall that the obtaining of a full account is delayed
until 24–48 hours has elapsed from the time of the initial report. The
statement should only be obtained by an officer who has undergone level 3
investigative interview training and who has an understanding of the trauma
surrounding such an incident. Several forces operate mentoring schemes
where less experienced officers shadow colleagues until they are comfortable
and confident in their own skills and abilities. However, this does need to be
balanced with the needs of the victim.

The location where the statement is obtained is important and, as
highlighted earlier in the chapter, many forces now have access to specialist
facilities. The surroundings, the time and support given and the demeanour
of the officer go a long way to assisting the victim in what is a very difficult
situation. There should be opportunities to take regular breaks, refreshments
should be available and most importantly the room should be located so that
it is free from interruption or other distractions. Recognition has been given
to the importance of video recording the interview with victims of serious
sexual assault. Officers trained in this technique will obtain a victim's
statement using this method.

The sexual offences liaison officer, as the name suggests, maintains
contact with the victim throughout the investigative process and beyond, if
the case is going through the judicial process. The sexual offences liaison
officer must be aware of their own limitations but more importantly the
expertise that is available via partner agencies such as Victim Support and
dedicated counselling and support services available.

In the HMCPSI/HMIC joint inspection into the investigation and
prosecution of cases involving allegations of rape, one of the major sources
of complaint was that victims were not kept informed of the progress of their
case, particularly when it entered the Criminal Justice System. Victims need

to be aware of timescales, the progress of the case and the position regarding the offender. This is important, as the victim has a genuine fear of reprisal if the offender is to be released from custody pending a court appearance. The victim needs to be aware of this and an appropriate safety plan discussed, which may include a personal attack alarm and additional security measures such as additional lights, good-quality locks, burglar alarm system or other security devices, and increased contact with a liaison officer.

Attending court

Significant progress has been made regarding the care of victims and witnesses throughout the criminal justice process. This gradual awareness of victim needs was highlighted in the 1996 Victim's Charter[7] and was emphasised in the work undertaken by the Home Office in *Speaking Up For Justice*[8] and *Action For Justice*,[9] which made a number of key recommend-ations putting victims and witnesses at the heart of the Criminal Justice System. Many of the recommendations within the reports were embodied in the Youth Justice and Criminal Evidence Act of 1999 and include the provision of special measures for certain categories of victims and witnesses which will be explored under the section headed 'New initiatives'. Many practical steps can be taken to support victims of rape and sexual assault, including contact with the witness service, which can give practical support including visiting the court to familiarise the individual with the layout of the building and practical information regarding the judicial processes. The most important aspect is that the victim is kept informed at every stage throughout the criminal justice process and is given relevant and up to date information to help prepare them to attend court.

For some witnesses, attendance at court may be a cathartic release: an opportunity to give their account and to have some form of closure in order to move forward. However, most victims view the court as an ordeal to be endured and have very real concerns around attending court, giving evidence and actually facing the perpetrator and associates. To minimise exposure to the perpetrator and/or associates, many courts have separate waiting facilities and some operate a pager system where the witness can wait in a neutral area away from the court and be paged when they are required to attend. The sexual offences liaison officer has a key role to perform in supporting the victim throughout and acting as a conduit with other agencies who can offer continuing support.

New initiatives

Research carried out by the Home Office into the treatment of vulnerable and intimidated witnesses highlighted that the current court processes were not allowing witnesses in rape or serious assault cases the opportunity to give their best evidence. This was highlighted in the research documents

Speaking Up For Justice[8] and *Action For Justice*.[9] As a result of this research, The Youth Justice and Criminal Evidence Act of 1999 was enacted, which allows special measures to be considered for certain categories of witnesses, including victims of rape or sexual assault. Also covered within the legislation are victims who are vulnerable because of age or disability or who are especially intimidated, which may include those subject to continuing domestic abuse.

For many years, child witnesses involved in sexual offences or abuse have had the opportunity to give their evidence in chief by a video recorded statement. The Youth Justice and Criminal Evidence Act 1999 expands upon this and allows other victims (vulnerable or intimidated) to be afforded the same treatment. This, together with other special measures, is intended to enable vulnerable and intimidated witnesses to give their best evidence in criminal proceedings.

It is well documented that many victims of sexual assault and rape find the experience of giving evidence in court not only stressful but also see it as a further violation and a continuation of the attack. The resultant stress undoubtedly impacts upon the quality of the communication between the victim and the court processes. Allowing victims the opportunity to give their evidence in chief by way of a pre-recorded video will ease some of the burden and lead to better presentation of evidence.

While the above is one of the more significant changes which impact upon victims of rape, a number of other measures are available which include the availability of screens that shield the witness from the defendant. Another groundbreaking initiative is the provision of a 'live link' to the courtroom. This enables the witness to give evidence from another room at the court via a televised link to the courtroom, thus reducing the trauma. This can be developed further, where the witness can be in a completely separate building and give evidence via live link. This will have a significant impact on those vulnerable witnesses who are hospitalised or have limited mobility. The live link has been used successfully from the home of an older person who had little or no mobility, in a case against a bogus official. Clearly, there is significant scope for this link to be considered for rape victims.

Other provisions under the Act include the removal of wigs by the judge and barrister to create a less intimidating atmosphere. At the request of the judge, members of the press and public, with the exception of one named person to represent the press, can be removed from the court in order that the victim's evidence can be given in private.

Numerous other special measures are available under the Act, which is viewed as the most far-reaching piece of legislation in offering support to victims and witnesses within the criminal justice system, while ensuring that the rights of the individual to a fair trial are not compromised. It must be stressed that such special measures are also available to defence witnesses if they also fulfil the criteria of vulnerable or intimidated witnesses who have identified special needs.

Special measures are not automatically granted but are subject to application by the prosecution prior to the trial. At the present time, the measures are currently being phased in and not all magistrates' courts have facilities that enable special measures to be adopted. All crown courts are currently reviewing provision to ensure they can comply with the legislation. It is clear that the criminal justice system has recognised that victims of crime, especially rape victims, need a comprehensive support mechanism to ensure that the evidence presented is the best they can give. It is envisaged that the measures that are being put in place will encourage victims of crime to come forward and to have faith in the criminal justice system. It is also hoped that the measure will assist the prosecution in increasing the number of successful prosecutions thus narrowing the justice gap.

References and notes

1. HM Crown Prosecution Service Inspectorate, HM Inspectorate of Constabulary. *A Report on the Joint Inspection into the Investigation and Prosecution of Cases Involving Allegations of Rape*. London: HMCPSI; April 2002. [www.homeoffice.gov.uk/hmic/CPSI_HMIC_Rape_Thematic.pdf].

2. REACH (Rape Examination Advice Counselling Help) opened in September 1991 to provide a free, confidential counselling, support and advice service for women (aged 16 years and over) who have been subjected to an attack of a sexual nature. It was initiated by Northumbria Police and their Women Doctors' Scheme to respond to clients' needs. Since 1 January 1998, REACH has been able to extend its remit of the service to include men aged 16 years and over. The service is available to people living in the Northumberland or Tyne and Wear areas, whether or not they make a formal complaint to the police.

3. St Mary's Sexual Assault Referral Centre, St Mary's Hospital, Hathersage Road, Manchester M13 0JH; telephone: 0161 276 6515; fax: 0161 276 6691; email: sarc@central.cmht.nwest.nhs.uk. The St Mary's Sexual Assault Referral Centre was established in 1986 and was the first of its kind in the UK, providing a comprehensive and coordinated forensic, counselling and medical aftercare service to adults in Greater Manchester who have been raped or sexually assaulted. The centre operates an open referral system on a 24-hour basis, whereby clients are able to access the full range of services without reporting to the police. The St Mary's Centre is situated in a specially designed suite of rooms within St Mary's Hospital, Manchester.

4. Juniper Lodge Sexual Assault Response Centre, Lodge 1, Leicestershire General Hospital, Gwedden Road, Leicester LE5 4PW; telephone & fax: 0116 273 5461; 24-hour help line: 0116 273 3330. Juniper Lodge opened in May 1999 to provide multi-agency support to survivors of rape and sexual assault in Leicestershire. The service offers an appropriate environment for examination for forensic evidence, statement taking and support work, whether or not clients wish police involvement. Telephone support, face-to-face counselling, information from specially trained police officers or a medical examination is offered to all clients. The Lodge is a dedicated centre that is fully furnished and decorated in a comfortable and non-threatening manner. It is located within the Leicester General Hospital Grounds in a convenient but discreet location.

5. The Haven, Caldecot Centre, London. 15–22 Caldecot Road, London SE5 9RS; telephone: 020 7346 1599. The Haven has been set up between the Metropolitan Police and King's College Hospital NHS Trust to provide comprehensive care for female and male complainants of sexual assault and rape. It aims to provide service users with a sensitive environment that can provide support about reporting to the police, the optimal collection of forensic and/or intelligence evidence (anonymously if desired); as well as being able to offer medical and psychosocial input. It can be accessed 24 hours a day, seven days a week by victims of sexual assault/rape themselves

or via the police. It is set in a self-contained unit within the sexual health department of King's College Hospital.

6. The REACH Centre, The Rhona Cross Centre, 18 Jesmond Road West, Newcastle Upon Tyne NE2 4PQ; telephone: 0191 212 1551; fax: 0191 212 1547; email: reach.newcastle@btinternet.com; or reach.sunderland@btinternet.com; website: www.reachcentre.org.uk. REACH (Rape, Examination, Advice, Counselling, Help) is a crisis intervention service, providing free, confidential, forensic medical examinations and/or short-term counselling and support for adults, regardless of whether they wish to report to the police. Both centres are comfortable and welcoming, with fully equipped medical examination suites, interview facilities and quiet rooms for counselling.

7. Home Office. Victim's Charter. [www.homeoffice.gov.uk/justice/victims/charter/index.html].

8. Home Office. *Speaking Up for Justice. Report of the Interdepartmental Working Group on the Treatment of Vulnerable or Intimidated Witnesses in the Criminal Justice System.* London: Home Office Procedures and Victims Unit; 1998.

9. Home Office. *Action for Justice. Implementing the Speaking Up for Justice Report on Vulnerable or Intimidated Witnesses in the Criminal Justice System in England and Wales.* London: Home Office Communication Directorate; 1999. [www.homeoffice.gov.uk/docs/actjust.pdf].

Appendix 2.1
Northumbria Police Training Unit Sexual Offences Liaison Officers Course

Rape is the most serious survivable crime. The treatment afforded to the victims of rape throughout the investigation process is key to the prospects of securing a conviction. Victims should be treated professionally, with respect and in accordance with their needs.

AIM

To prepare the officer for the role of a Sexual Offences Liaison Officer (SOLO) by building on their existing skills and abilities.

LEARNING OUTCOMES

Understand the role of a SOLO, the need to support and guide the victim through the investigation process. Liaise with the investigation team and access the full services of REACH. Have the required knowledge to obtain an initial account from the victim.

CRITERIA

Has completed two-year probation. Is PEACE interview trained, has attended a two-day Northumbria Police diversity course and is a qualified police driver.

PROGRAMME

Discussed on the course are matters relating to rape and other serious sexual assaults on men and women. Practical techniques are used in the training and students are asked to take an active role. The course is intense and reflects Northumbria Police Policy and guidance and the recommendations made in the HMCPSI/HMIC report on the joint investigation and prosecution of cases involving allegations of rape. Duration: three days.

Lesson: Role of the SOLO

Aim

To provide the students with an overview of the role performed by the SOLO.

Objectives

At the end of the session, the students will be able to:
1. define rape as per force policy
2. state the seven principles of the investigation
3. explain the role of the SOLO
4. summarise the elements of the role.

Lesson: Knowledge check on legislation

Aim

To provide the students with an opportunity to check their understanding of sexual offences legislation.

Objectives

At the end of the session, the students will be able to:
1. distinguish between an act of rape and indecent assault
2. identify when consent would never be true consent for rape and indecent assault
3. compare force policy in relation to rape with the current legislation.

Lesson: CID 9 – the SOLO log book

Aim

To provide the students with the knowledge to engage in the initial contact and complete a CID 9.

Objectives

At the end of the session, the students will be able to:
1. state the purpose of the CID 9
2. give examples of the contents required
3. demonstrate the completion of a CID 9
4. demonstrate the initial contact with the victim.

Lesson: Attitudes and values

Aim

To provide the students with the knowledge of how their judgement of a victim could affect the investigation.

Objectives

At the end of the session, the students will be able to:
1.   explain Betaris Box
2.   describe how values and attitudes are formed
3.   recognise the impact of the wrong attitude on the victim.

Lesson: Visit to REACH

Aim

To provide the students with knowledge of how to access REACH and its services.

Objectives

At the end of the session, the students will be able to:
1.   explain how to access the building 24 hours a day.
2.   outline the structure of the examination conducted by the doctor.
3.   summarise the methods used to obtain the samples.
4.   outline the reasons for the examination.
5.   describe the referral procedure for counselling.
6.   outline the role of the councillors.

Lesson: Practical and packaging

Aim

To demonstrate the packaging and recording of samples taken during a forensic medical examination.

Objectives

At the end of the session, the students will be able to:
1.   demonstrate how to identify, record and package samples handed over by the FME
2.   state what forms need to be completed
3.   summarise the information required on the forms
4.   describe the layout of both REACH centres.

Lesson: Drug rape

Aim

To provide the students with the knowledge to deal with a victim who has been drug raped.

Objectives

At the end of the session, the students will be able to:
1. explain how to use an early evidence urine kit
2. describe the effects of drug rape upon the victim
3. outline lines of initial investigation.

Lesson: Male rape

Aim

To provide the students with an understanding of the effects of rape on men.

Objectives

At the end of the session, the students will be able to:
1. recognise additional areas of anxiety for a male victim
2. explain support available.

Lesson: Rape trauma syndrome

Aim

To provide the students with knowledge of rape trauma syndrome and the effect this has on a victim's character and behaviour.

Objectives

At the end of the session, the students will be able to:
1. state the 3 stages of rape trauma syndrome.
2. summarise the feelings/fears/reactions a victim can experience.
3. give examples of how people can help the victim.

Lesson: Victim care

Aim

To provide the students with the knowledge to liaise effectively with the victim.

Objectives

At the end of the session, the students will be able to:
1. name the agencies involved with the support of the victim
2. explain the purpose of the Victim Personal Statement
3. describe the protocol of information
4. identify what information should be provided to the victim concerning the offender.

Lesson: Rape – paperfeed

Aim

To give the students an opportunity to consolidate their new knowledge by giving them an opportunity to discuss a number of issues raised in an investigation of rape. To provide an opportunity for the trainer to test the students' understanding of the SOLO's role.

Objectives

At the end of the session, the students will be able to:
1. analyse their ability to perform the role of SOLO, identifying areas that need developing.
2. recall all of the aspects that must be covered in the initial contact with the victim.
3. outline the procedure to be followed when calling out a doctor.
4. summarise the care that must be afforded to the victim.
5. identify an exit strategy.

Chapter 3

Avenues of presentation:
dilemmas facing medical practitioners when presented with cases of sexual assault

Mary Pillai

Introduction

There is no such thing as a typical victim or scenario of sexual assault. In most cases the victim knows the assailant. A high proportion of assaults occur in the victim's home or that of an acquaintence.[1] All age groups are affected but teenagers are by far the most vulnerable group.[2] Many offences are committed by a partner or ex-partner in the context of domestic abuse. The problem is not confined to women, however, although male complainants are very much in the minority. Three percent of men participating in a GP-based survey reported non-consensual sexual experiences as adults and 5% reported sexual abuse as children.[3] There are few data on whether men may be even less likely to make official complaints following sexual assault than women.

MacDonald highlighted the global picture of an estimated one in five women experiencing at least one episode of sexual assault or rape.[4] Health professionals in the UK have tended to ignore the fact that we also have this problem closer to home. The effects of the crime present to health professionals in the guise of a wide variety of medical problems. Part of the problem is the profession's reluctance to address sexual violence. Sexual violence is everyone's problem but no one's responsibility. The training needs of health professionals to respond to interpersonal and family violence have not been met so far in either the undergraduate curriculum or in specialist training, despite this problem accounting for more morbidity than many common health concerns.

Sexual assault in the UK

Current figures for sexual offences in England and Wales are summarised in Table 3.1.[5]

Although there has been a three-fold increase in the number of allegations of rape since 1985, research evidence indicates this still represents only a minority of cases. Significant factors militate against reporting an incident

Table 3.1 Sexual offences in England and Wales (*n*)[5]

Year	1997–98	1998–99	1999–2000	2000–01	2001–02
All sexual offences	34151	36174	37792	37299	41425
Rape:					
female			7809	7929	9008
male			600	664	735
Indecent assault:					
female			20664	20301	21765
male			3614	3530	3613
Buggery			437	401	354
Unlawful sexual intercourse:					
with a girl under 13 years			181	155	170
with a girl under 16 years			1270	1273	1336
Incest			121	80	93
Gross indecency with a child			1365	1336	1665

and making an official complaint. Consequently, establishing the exact number of offences is extremely difficult. Published data from the UK indicate that perhaps 22% of cases are reported,[5] while US data suggest that 19–28% of women who have been assaulted report these incidents to the police and other mainstream agencies.[2,6] Less than 7% of people contacting Rape Crisis had reported their assault to the police.[1] This is compounded by the fact that only a small percentage of reported cases proceed to court and few convictions are obtained (Table 3.2).

Among women who contact Rape Crisis, reported experience shows that:

- 97% knew their assailant
- the most common rapists are current or ex-partners
- one in seven married women said they had been forced to have sex compared with one in three divorced or separated women
- 91% of women had told no one.

Table 3.2 Attrition rate for rape cases in England and Wales (Home Office statistics)

Year	Reported cases (*n*)	Convictions (*n*)	Conviction rate (%)
1977	1015	324	32
1987	2471	453	18
1992	4142	410	10
1996	5759 (f); 231 (m)	573	10
2000	7809 (f); 600 (m)	–	7

Despite low reporting rates, there is evidence women are very concerned about the adverse effects on their health. Among women who were followed up, physical health consequences of pregnancy and sexually transmitted infections (STIs) were identified in a minority.[7] However, psychological sequelae were common and included disturbances of sleep, sexual function and appetite, and numerous assault-related fears.

Time of assault

A consistent pattern of assault is found in respect to both the time of day and day of the week, with a predominance between 6 p.m. and 6 a.m. (67%) and a peak occurring on Friday to Monday and the lowest risk day being Wednesday.[2] Presentation can be within hours or may be years after the attack.

Rape trauma syndrome

The literature is replete with studies showing common psychological symptoms, which together constitute what has been termed 'rape trauma syndrome'. Evidence of this has been admitted as scientific testimony in criminal trials.[8] This syndrome falls more widely under the umbrella term of post-traumatic stress disorder, for which sexual assault is one of many possible causes. Sexual assault has been reported to be the most common cause of post-traumatic stress disorder in American women.[9]

The *Diagnostic and Statistical Manual of Mental Disorders*, 4th edition, defines post-traumatic stress disorder as "the development of characteristic symptoms following exposure to an extreme traumatic stressor involving direct personal experience of an event that involves actual or threatened death or serious injury, or other threat to one's physical integrity".[10] Symptoms must be present for at least one month and include persistent re-experiencing of the event, avoidance of stimuli associated with the event and increased arousal. For many victims, hypervigilance towards most men may be permanent. There must also be an accompanying impairment in social, occupational or other important realm of functioning. These emotional, cognitive and physiological reactions that are experienced by people exposed to any traumatic event may be experienced for weeks, months or even years after the event. They do not necessarily represent an unhealthy or maladaptive response but rather a normal response to an abnormal event.

Although post-traumatic stress disorder is common following sexual assault, there is no evidence that brief psychological debriefing reduces this.[11] At present, there are insufficient data on how to best address this, but it is agreed good practice to offer information about rape crisis groups and any other local victim support service.

Factors that influence presentation

There are significant deficiencies in the service that individuals who make a complaint are likely to receive, with no consistency nationwide. In many areas, examination suites are based in police premises, with deficient facilities for contamination control and dependence upon doctors who are otherwise engaged in full-time work. This means that the forensic examination may be significantly delayed, due to searching for an available doctor or a gap in a busy clinical schedule. The examination gathers forensic evidence but rarely addresses health issues beyond emergency contraception. Most areas do not offer prophylaxis or any follow-up for other health consequences. Instead, complainants are directed to make their own appointments in mainstream genitourinary services in competition with general patients seeking screening and treatment for sexual infections. This is far removed from the ideal of a comprehensive medical and forensic service of the highest quality, where an examination, evidence collection and appropriate health interventions can occur while the complainant is undecided about involving the criminal justice system.

The legal system has traditionally discriminated against women and the judicial system has offered little protection. Within relationships, women are far less likely to complain about episodes of forced sexual activity. "The greater the degree of social relationship, the wider the latitude of permitted coercion, so that an act of forced sex committed by a stranger may be recognised as rape, while the same act committed by a partner is not."[12] Only since 1994 has the UK legal system accepted that rape can take place in marriage. In 1995, all countries belonging to the United Nations voted in Beijing to abolish the marital privilege to sex on demand from wives.

Admitting to having been raped remains one of the major social taboos. The anonymous writer of a moving personal view clearly describes the effects of such taboos, of keeping private "the shameful secret" of having been raped: "It was as if I had a chronic abscess inside … sapping all my strength and energy".[13] Victims also fear the process of examination, which of itself may be perceived as a further violation. However, the most formidable prospect of all is often having to relive the experience in a court process, where attempts will be made to discredit their name and reputation. A further disincentive is the low likelihood of securing a conviction.[14] The percentage of court cases that secured a conviction for rape fell dramatically between 1977 and 2000 (Table 3.2), and a report on drug-assisted rape cited a conviction rate as low as 6%.[15]

Terminology

Many terms have been used for individuals who claim or are believed to have suffered sexual assault: 'victim', 'survivor' and 'patient' are probably most common. However, the term 'complainant' is more appropriate for forensic purposes in that it does not presume what has happened. This may not be so appropriate in other settings, for which the broader term 'client' has been advocated as being neutral and recognising the initial and continuing relationships the person has with healthcare and other professionals.[16]

Where complainants present

Although presentation may be in the context of a direct complaint to the police, because of low reporting, probably more cases present to health professionals in the guise of health problems or anxiety either at the time or, more usually, at some later date. Thus, presentation will span a range of services. The most common will include accident and emergency, genito-urinary medicine, gynaecology, family planning and pregnancy termination services, GP, rape crisis or other counselling services and psychiatric services. Seeking medical help can be traumatic for victims, who may feel they are being violated all over again by the examination.

Police complaints

The majority of forensic examinations follow a direct complaint to the police. A long period of waiting while an examination is arranged, during which they are asked not to wash, adds further distress to their experience. Currently, most forensic examinations take place in police premises and, apart from emergency contraception, do not include health issues for the complainant. For these health concerns, complainants are directed to other services but evidence supports the fact that take up is minimal.[7,17]

Characteristics of complainants

Although extremes of age are included, the majority of complainants are teenagers or young adults (Table 3.3). The risk peaks in the late teens, with girls aged 16–19 years being four times more likely to be assaulted or raped than the rest of the population. Most incidents occur during high-risk behaviour and most involve considerable quantities of alcohol.

Vulnerability factors are listed in Table 3.4. Vulnerability may be by age or learning disability, or it may be due to family factors such as abusive relationships or young people with inappropriate and inconsistent boundaries.

Abusive relationships may be part of a self-perpetuating lifestyle. Both men and women with a past history of abuse have low self-esteem and often have low expectations of how they will be treated in a relationship, which leaves them vulnerable to adult relationships of control and disrespect. It is common that families in which abuse occurs are socially isolated. Social isolation does not simply happen. There is often a pattern of jealous surveillance of all social contacts, which limits any opportunity for

Table 3.3 Percentage of sexual assault or rape by age of victim (US Bureau of Justice)[6]

Age group (years)	Cases (%)
Under 12	15
12–17	29
Under 18	44
Under 30	80

maintaining normal friendships and socialising outside the family. This behaviour by the abuser preserves the needed secrecy and control over family members.

The elderly

Older female rape victims are more likely to live alone, to be raped by strangers, to experience physical force or injury and to be robbed.[18] Those who suffer in residential accommodation tend to be those with mental incapacity, especially dementia. The extremes of age often have in common that victims cannot make the complaint themselves and it is made on their behalf by a third party. An appropriate adult must always accompany individuals with impaired ability when a forensic examination is requested.

Table 3.4 Vulnerability factors for sexual assault

Vulnerability factor	Risks
Social competence	Young age
	Incompetent by way of illness, e.g. Alzheimer's disease or head injury
	Naïve due to learning disability
	Psychiatric disorder (especially in adolescence)
Alcohol	Large quantities are involved in 70–80% of cases
	Drugs (less common)
Risk taking behaviour	Unsafe company
	Walking or accepting lift home with new acquaintance/s
	Allowing someone not well known into house when alone
	Experimenting with alcohol and drugs
Children with vulnerable lifestyle	Lack of age-appropriate boundaries, e.g. young teens clubbing late at night
	Children in care
	Children running away, vulnerable to exploitation
Abusive relationships	Domestic violence frequently includes sexual violence
	Lack of family support
	Social isolation
	Low self-esteem with lack of expectation about how they will be treated

CASE A

A request was made to conduct a forensic examination on an 83-year-old lady with Alzheimer's disease. The superintendent of the care home where she lived made the complaint. Two members of staff found evidence of a forced entry and encountered a young man fleeing from her room with his trousers undone. She was on the floor with her incontinence pad removed. The woman was not capable of giving consent to a forensic examination. A dilemma of consent was posed. No one can give consent to examination or treatment of another person over the age of 18 years, regardless of loss of their own ability to consent. In this circumstance, the next of kin was consulted and a decision made to proceed with the examination on two counts. Firstly, the relatives believed that if the woman were still able to consent she would want the examination. Secondly, there was a public interest issue. It was therefore agreed that, provided she did not resist or become distressed by the examination, it should take place. There were fresh superficial injuries to her back and limbs, compatible with her having been dragged out of bed on to the floor. There was a tear to the posterior fourchette area. Further examination of the vagina was not possible, as she became distressed. Forensic swabs from the appropriate area did provide important evidential evidence in this case.

For practical reasons the examination in this case took place in the care home but this is not ideal. As a minimum, a good light source is essential and the specimens must be collected, sealed and signed in a forensically sound method.

Adolescents

Teenagers are the highest risk group for sexual assault, with approximately one-third of all reports involving this age group and 25% involving those under 16 years (Table 3.3). Among adolescents, young people in the care system are at highest risk, reflecting a risky life style. There is also a complex interrelationship with psychiatric co-morbidity. Studies from New Zealand[19] have found a clear association between risky sexual behaviour and common psychiatric disorders. Young people with depression, substance dependence, antisocial personality, mania and the schizophrenia spectrum are all more likely to engage in risky sexual behaviour and to contract sexually transmitted infection.[19] Although the temporal relation is uncertain, the results indicate the need to coordinate sexual medicine with mental health services in the treatment of young people.

It is well recognised that inconsistent and inappropriate boundaries render young people highly vulnerable. Risk taking is common but, at the same time, they are less likely to have acquired the social skills to recognise or disengage themselves from situations of danger. It may be that the coexistence of psychiatric morbidity further impairs the mechanisms that keep young people safe when they take risks.

Risky behaviour and omnipotence of the peer group may lead young teenagers to believe they should have sex but with no expectation of how they will be treated. Physical violence is relatively common in teen dating and young teens tend to romanticise jealousy. This perpetuates a culture of disrespect, particularly for women. Another study of young people in New Zealand[20] found that only 0.2% of young men but 7% of women reported being forced to have intercourse on the first occasion. For women, there were increasing rates of coercion with younger age at first intercourse. Most women regretted having sexual intercourse before the age of 16 years. First intercourse at younger ages is associated with risks that are shared unequally between men and women. This information is important to young people themselves.

Sexual health concerns bring young people into contact with health services and this provides an opportunity to screen for problems. However, it is a considerable challenge to know how best to engage young people in 'keep safe' work. For example, one can enquire if sex was enjoyed and wanted, whether they have any concerns, whether their boyfriend is ever violent or jealous and whether they have felt pressured to have sex. If one is perceived to be judgemental they will not use the service again. However, if provided with an opportunity to talk about their experience in a safe, unpressured environment, a significant number of young girls seeking emergency contraception do reveal that the episode was not only unprotected but was unwanted and not enjoyed. This provides the best opportunity for discussing preventive strategies. In most cases of this nature, a formal complaint to the police is never an issue and would not be helpful.

A number of complaints arise where the alleged victim did not know what had happened to them or whether anything had happened, particularly among adolescents. Either the girl or a third party suspected that a sexual assault may have been perpetrated on the basis of being heavily under the influence of alcohol (or occasionally drugs) and remembering partial events, waking unclothed or what a friend reported seeing (Case B). Occasionally, there was suspicion of drugs being given without consent, usually by means of drink. In many such cases an assumption is made by the complainant that a forensic examination can tell what has happened and, often, this is the main motivation for reporting the assault to the police. However, it rarely turns out that forensic examination can help, as most times an examination is inconclusive. Occasionally, there are findings but most often these are nonspecific and not confirmatory of a criminal event. Evidence of semen either on clothing from the incident or swabs may be found by the forensic laboratory but is rarely obvious on the forensic examination itself.

Date rape

Also referred to as 'acquaintance rape' and 'hidden rape', this accounts for a much greater number of cases than has previously been acknowledged. The work of psychologist Mary Koss has informed the scope and severity of

CASE B

The mother of a thirteen-year-old girl informed the police that she wished to make a complaint of possible rape against her daughter. The girl had been at an outdoor party. She remembered drinking a considerable quantity of alcohol but could not remember events thereafter. Her friends reported that a boy took her into a tent and closed it. Later she was found asleep in the tent. The bottom half of her clothes had been removed. The girl reported that she was not sexually active and not using any medication. She felt sore and had noted some stinging when passing urine. Examination revealed no external or genital injuries. The hymen was of the fimbriated type and it was impossible to say whether penetration might have occurred. Swabs were taken and levonorgestrel prescribed as a precautionary measure. In view of the lack of any substantive finding or complaint the case was not pursued so the forensic samples were never analysed.

the problem, debunking the belief that unwanted sexual advances and intercourse were not rape if they occurred with an acquaintance or on a date.[21–23]

Any form of coercion, be it menacing pressure, use of drugs or alcohol, or misuse of authority, undermines consent and renders the resulting sexual activity unlawful. Self-esteem plays an important role in how young people expect to be treated within relationships. It is essential that vulnerable people understand that they do not owe it to anyone to have sex and especially not because that person has paid for the date or done something for them. Other myths that surround date rape include:

- a girl who gets raped usually deserves it, especially if she agreed to go to the man's house or park with him or invited him into her house
- certain behaviours, such as drinking or dressing in a sexually appealing way, make rape a woman's responsibility
- intimate kissing or certain kinds of touching mean that intercourse is inevitable
- once a man reaches a certain point of arousal, sex is inevitable and they can't help forcing themselves on women
- most women lie about acquaintance rape because they have regrets about consensual sex
- women who don't fight back haven't been raped.

These beliefs are common, and provide a general disincentive to making an official complaint. Women are significantly less likely to go to the police about date rape than a stranger assault, and often blame themselves for not seeing it coming before it was too late. This may unwittingly be reinforced by family, friends and professionals, in the form of questioning their decision to drink during a date or to invite the assailant back for coffee.

Many women do not put up resistance through fear and in the instance that no resistance is offered there will usually be no abnormal forensic findings. Where the defence claim consent, forensic testing is not likely to be of value but careful documentation of bodily injuries may provide key evidence. However, in the author's experience, even the presence of multiple injuries in a distribution that could not be self-inflicted may not convince a jury that the girl did not consent. This poses a considerable dilemma for the Crown Prosecution Service, whose guidelines for criminal prosecution are that the case must be beyond reasonable doubt. For civil proceedings, as with Family Court or child protection cases, the lesser standard of balance of probability is required.

Who commits acquaintance rape?

Acquaintance rape is not typically committed by psychopaths who are deviant from mainstream society. Young people are bombarded with messages portraying sex as a commodity whose attainment is the ultimate male challenge: "I'm going to make it tonight", "I'm going to score with her". Messages given to boys and young men about what it means to be male (dominant, aggressive, uncompromising) contribute to creating a mindset which is accepting of sexually aggressive behaviour. It is therefore not surprising that typically the perpetrator and the victim have very different perceptions of what happened. One in twelve male US college students surveyed had committed acts that met the legal definition of rape or attempted rape but 84% of those who had committed rape said that what they did was definitely not rape.[22] Male perpetrators have a strong inclination to normalise events and think that it is quite acceptable to use force when needed. Many men use rape myths and false stereotypes about 'what women really want' to rationalise sexually aggressive behaviour. Typical statements include "She said no, but she really meant yes". The most widely used defence is to blame the victim and, in most cases, this includes that the girl consented. It is difficult to prove consent or not in alleged date rape.

Multiple perpetrators and gang rapes

In most rapes there is a single perpetrator. However, 16% of male students who committed rape and 10% of those who attempted rape took part in episodes involving more than one attacker.[22]

Sometimes, the perpetrator is aided by others who forcibly restrain the victim. In the instance that a person has aided a rape, they also can be charged with the rape, even when they did not engage in sexual contact. In this circumstance, women can be charged with rape together with men.

Gang rape is reported to be common in some cultures and in some UK inner cities but it is rare in rural areas. It may form part of a gang 'initiation'.

Drug-assisted rape

Excluding alcohol, other drugs are associated with a minority of sexual assault complaints in the UK. The Sturman report has evaluated drug-assisted sexual assault and made detailed recommendations to the Home Office.[15] No one drug alone is responsible. Between four and five different drugs are being used to commit this offence, often in conjunction with alcohol, which heightens the reaction. Interviews with complainants revealed that 70% of attacks were committed by acquaintances with 80% of those questioned having some memory of the incident. Drugs such as flunitrazepam (Rohypnol®, Roche) and gamma hydroxybutyrate (GHB) are tasteless, colourless and odourless, as well as being cheap, and thus easily administered by addition to a drink. They have potent amnesic, hypnotic and disinhibitory effects.

CASE C

A 25-year-old woman presented to the pregnancy advisory service with a request for termination. She was distressed about the circumstances of the pregnancy, in that she had no partner and did not know who was responsible for the pregnancy. Some weeks earlier she had been to a club with a friend and there they met up with a group of young men, some of whom were known to them. One of the group that they had not met before invited them to go back to a party. She remembered going but could not remember anything else. The friend told her she had a few drinks with the man and then disappeared into one of the bedrooms with him. Thinking she had gone voluntarily, the friend decided to go home. The next thing the woman remembered was waking up on the couch in her own flat but she did not know how she got there. Later, she contacted the friend and was alarmed by the events she reported. When her next period did not come and a pregnancy test was positive she went to the police and made a complaint. The dilemma here was that by then it was too late to take forensic samples and there was insufficient evidence to pursue the case or find the suspect. The woman was keen for forensic DNA evidence to be collected at the termination. This can be done only if arrangements are made for any tissue to be collected in a manner that ensures the chain of evidence. Another issue is the cost of testing, which would need to be agreed with the police, since it would not be the responsibility of the health trust. This sort of forensic analysis is costly and would not be authorised unless there was a reasonable prospect it would lead to a conviction.

Domestic assault

The term 'domestic' is taken to mean between individuals in a family-type relationship, wherever the violence occurs. A study of Coventry in 1995 found that, in that year alone, the proportion of women known to the police as victims of domestic violence amounted to 1.25% of all adult women residents.[24] Both men and women experience domestic violence, although predominantly it is women who are the victims (96% versus 4% of victims being men). The majority of repetitive assaults are carried out by men against their female partner, although abuse does on rare occasions occur in same-sex relationships. The issue centres on an abuse of power and control, usually involving a pattern that becomes more severe over time and often involves alcohol and sexual abuse.

Intimate partner violence has many wide-ranging sequelae, including adverse pregnancy outcomes. It affects 3–13% of pregnancies in studies from around the world and is associated with detrimental outcomes to both mothers and infants.[25]

For an affected woman, there are considerable disincentives to reporting domestic violence, including the anticipated response of the authorities that might render her situation even more difficult.[26] Professionals relied upon for support are not immune to subtly blaming the woman. For example, they may ask what she did to provoke the incident, why she does not leave or why she allows it to happen. They may fail to acknowledge the woman's need for safety by avoiding asking whether it is safe for her to return home or whether she has somewhere else to go if the violence escalates. Even if doctors do ask, they are usually at a loss to know how to respond. They have inadequate knowledge of available local refuges or how to make contact on the woman's behalf. Most could offer an NHS bed overnight and then rely on social services.

False allegations

It is not known what proportion of complaints of sexual violence may arise from false claims. A false claim is easy to make but it is virtually impossible to counter, since one cannot prove a negative. The absence of substantive evidence is common in forensic examinations but is not generally given weight or taken as evidence that rape or molestation did not happen. Sometimes an agenda is clarified. On review of cases in Gloucestershire over a 12-month period, at least two cases were clarified as false and a third impossible. In one case, a 14-year-old claimed a stranger assault. There were no findings and an inconsistent story. She later admitted the claim was to appease her parents when she went home very late. In the second case, a 29-year-old woman claimed stranger assault by two men. Her past history aroused suspicion and it was later established the motive was to avert a domestic situation, having left her husband baby-sitting for considerably longer than had been agreed. In the third case, allegations by a severely disturbed young woman were so numerous, extreme and sexually violent that the normal genital findings and intact oestrogen-deficient hymen precluded any possibility the claims could be real, although the young woman appeared sincere in believing the events. There was evidence that, over time, her allegations had been incremental and, as the story grew, the details had become more violent and bizarre (Case E).

There are considerable pressures on professionals and agencies to respond to all complaints of sexual assault with support and empathy. Conversely, little publicity and sympathy is attracted by victims of false reporting. There is no robust means by which false claims can be recognised. The apparent distress of the victim is not a good guide to reliability. A study evaluating the viability of rape trauma syndrome in alleged rape cases found that rape cases did score higher than controls but those who faked rape endorsed a greater number of symptoms than actual rape victims. False claims were also associated with a greater number of fictitious and unlikely symptoms.[27] The study concluded that evaluation of a symptom score might be of some value in ascertaining the veracity of claims where circumstances are equivocal.

Claims generate a great deal of attention and have considerable consequences. Where claims are made relating to children in the context of a custody dispute, extreme caution is needed. Children are especially vulnerable to believing what they hear from a trusted adult and, in this situation, may repeatedly be given information of a negative type about one or other parent.[28] During protracted investigation of such cases, it is common for children to be denied access to one of their parents, usually the father, for many months or years. Where the allegation was false, this of itself is an extreme emotional abuse of the child. Although uncommon, there have been cases of mothers making allegations about their children and other people, as a way of gaining attention, and seemingly disregarding the trauma the resulting investigation and assessments will cause for the child.[29]

Unfounded allegations may occasionally come from relatives, neighbours, teachers and other professionals but usually they will have been made in good faith. The harm done to those falsely accused is considerable.[30] It parallels the harm suffered by unrecognised genuine cases and, for these reasons, a balance needs to be achieved.

Presentation in clinical practice

Victims may reveal that they have been attacked immediately, a few days, months or even years later. Each clinical area where a victim may disclose acutely or within a few days needs to have a clear understanding and protocol of management. When complainants present after sexual assault to a health professional in the short term, a sensitive enquiry should be made as to whether they have reported to the police or would like to. In this circumstance, examination is a medico-legal emergency, as most positive evidence will be dissipated by 72 hours. Forensic examination should be considered a possible source of useful evidence for up to seven days after an assault, especially if semen has been deposited in the vagina. Where possible, the forensic examination must be performed prior to any medical examination. If a complainant requests police involvement then the local police control room should be notified immediately and no further history or examination performed until after any forensic examination.

A recognised long-term consequence of sexual assault is the perception of ill health. As a direct concern arising from the event, 20% of women who have been sexually assaulted use medical services in the first year, rising to 50% in the second year.[7] The most common delayed presentations are chronic pain syndrome, lowered self-perception of health and self-harming behaviour.

It is most unfortunate that medical training has only in recent times included psychosocial factors and, so far, has not included management of sexual and other relationship violence. Doctors whose work is hospital-based are particularly distant from a holistic view of patients' health needs within their environmental context. There is little opportunity to observe or understand the patient's perspective. Williamson has identified multiple problems relating to the way in which healthcare professionals interact with patients who have experienced domestic violence, undermining the contribution they may be able to make.[26] These shortcomings are more widely applicable to all sexual violence.

Injuries

Significant physical injury from a sexual assault is rare and it is exceptional that injuries result in the need for hospitalisation. The absence of injuries proves a lack of force but it does not prove consent.

Significant injury is more common in stranger attacks and rapes by a domestic partner. In domestic violence, the injuries tend to be inflicted where the victim can most easily hide them. Injury is also more common in male victims. Intentional injuries tend to be central, while accidental injuries are towards the extremities.

Not all women who have been sexually assaulted have visible genital injury. No evidence of trauma at all was found in 20% of cases in one large study.[17] Generalised injuries are more common than genital trauma, especially if resistance has been offered.[17,31]

Miller et al.[32] studied the characteristics of cases where immediate help was sought versus delay in presentation. The severity of attack prompted women to seek treatment earlier but also women who were assaulted by a stranger were much more likely to seek immediate assistance than those assaulted by a known perpetrator.

The accident and emergency department

When there are serious physical injuries, complainants will most often present to the accident and emergency department or will be taken there by the police. Treatment of serious injuries takes precedence over any collection of forensic evidence. If clothing needs to be removed, care should be taken to avoid cutting through damaged areas, such as rips, tears or stab holes. It is important to take samples of blood and urine as soon as it is reasonable to do so, to avoid evidence being lost with time. These samples may subsequently be admissible as evidence, provided that they have been collected and handled in an evidentially sound manner (see Chapter 8). If the complainant does not wish to make a complaint to the police then whoever deals with them should take a comprehensive history and carefully document the examination findings. This information may subsequently be requested as evidence but should not be disclosed without signed consent from the client or by order of the Court.

The genitourinary medicine service

Clinical guidelines have been issued for complainants presenting to genitourinary medicine clinics.[33] Gonorrhoea, chlamydia and trichomoniasis are the sexually transmitted infections most frequently identified in women who give a history of sexual assault.[34,35] It is desirable that a full screen for sexually transmitted infections is undertaken at presentation, as there is a significant incidence of pre-existing infection among women who allege rape.

A pragmatic and compassionate approach is needed. The benefit to the patient must be weighed against exacerbating or prolonging her distress. In situations where the patient may default or decline initial or repeat examination, consideration should be given to antibiotic prophylaxis. There is a case that all sexual assault complainants should be offered the choice of antimicrobial prophylaxis, as many would choose this in preference to, or in addition to, follow-up screening.

The obstetrics and gynaecology service

The climate of a painfully disrupted sexual history or on-going abusive relationship may generate many presentations. These may be:

- commented on in the GP referral letter
- disclosed by the patient during the course of consultation
- disclosed when difficulties arise with intimate examination
- presented as chronic pelvic pain with no organic cause
- presented as sexual dysfunction:
  - dyspareunia and apareunia (pain can be an avoidance mechanism)
  - loss or lack of libido
  - vaginismus
  - a request for assisted conception because sex unacceptable
- presented as an unwanted pregnancy
- a request for elective caesarean section because of the unacceptability of vaginal examination or vaginal delivery.

CASE D

A 29-year-old woman had originally been referred with longstanding depression and premenstrual symptoms some five years earlier. She had been treated with antidepressants and homeopathic remedies by her GP. She took up the option of a Mirena® (Schering Health) intrauterine system (IUS) and persisted with this for almost four years. This had minimised her bleeding and made her cycle difficult to determine but she said this had only made her severe mood swings worse. These were now characterised by unprovoked outbursts of shouting and threats towards her children. The IUS had been removed four months earlier, because she wanted a cycle again. Now the referral was marked urgent because she was "unable to cope". She reported severe symptoms lasting for three weeks out of four. She was not prepared to take tablets any more and wanted a hysterectomy. She had read that this was a good treatment and couldn't understand why it hadn't been offered.

Attempts to explore the possibility that perhaps the emotional outbursts needed to be viewed more in the context of what else was happening in her life were rejected. Explanation that data did not support hysterectomy as an effective treatment prompted hostility and so it was suggested that another opinion might be the best way forward. Her anger increased and after stating that her right to this choice should override professional difficulty with it, she left the clinic abruptly. It was anticipated that a complaint might follow. Instead, some five weeks later an urgent referral for termination arrived. The pregnancy was already 16 weeks but she said she had been having bleeds and so had not considered she might be pregnant. She did not bring up the previous conversation. Sensitive enquiry about her partner's reaction to the pregnancy led to a disclosure of a longstanding relationship of violence and abuse. Under no circumstances did she wish him to know of the pregnancy. She went on to talk about the hopelessness of having another child in her situation. Discussion centred on the role of the domestic violence unit and the safety of her children as well as her own immediate and long-term needs and the options available to her.

This young woman's request for hysterectomy may have held many agendas and, not least, an element of self-destruction in the midst of a cycle of abuse and control. Patients do not have the right to demand treatment that the doctor does not believe to be indicated on medical grounds. Moreover, doctors have a duty of care to prevent patients doing things to themselves that are harmful and, particularly, to avoid collusion with drastic measures that are not supported by evidence.

Conversely, doctors should be cautious about forming conclusions that a sexual difficulty indicates likely abuse. A study of the prevalence of physical or sexual violence among women referred with vulval dysaesthesia compared with controls in a general clinic found no relationship with sexual assault.[36] However, where interpersonal relationship problems are present, the sexual issues will likely prove resistant to intervention while the woman continues in an abusive relationship. This is especially true when the woman is presenting on behalf of her partner who wants the problem 'sorted'. Picking up the signals that something is wrong and asking appropriate questions takes considerable sensitivity and skill, which hitherto has not been included in gynaecological training. This approach is essential if inappropriate investigations, such as laparoscopy, are to be avoided and the woman helped to face the problem constructively and to explore the options available to her.

Even if the woman is in a new relationship free of any abuse, the problem may still be difficult to manage. Satisfaction drives interest and is unlikely to be derived against a background of associating sex with control and violation. Some women may present challenging symptoms that are both extreme and refractory, leading to inappropriate requests for drastic measures.

Interviewing strategies

Doctors have a natural reluctance to ask patients about intimate violence but failure to do so when this may be an issue makes diagnosis difficult and precludes appropriate advice and support. Appropriate questions require the right moment and should, where possible, be open-ended; for example:

Q: "How often do you feel like sex?"
A: "Not at all"
Q: "Have you ever felt obliged or coerced?"
A: "Yes"
Q: "And what happens if you say you don't want to……"

or

"I notice that you have a number of bruises. Could you tell me how that happened?"

Research has shown that women are more likely to report abuse and violence when questioned sensitively by a health provider, compared with filling out an anonymous questionnaire.[37]

Paediatric presentations

Child sexual abuse

Presentations of sexual abuse in children are varied and may include:

- symptoms disclosed by the child
- abuse suspected by a parent or carer

- evidence of other forms of abuse
- symptoms due to anogenital injury
- sexually transmitted infection
- exposure to a known abuser
- examination requested by police or social services as part of an investigation or ordered by the Court to assist with care proceedings
- suspected on the basis of abuse to other children in the family or in the same care circumstance coming to light
- a wide range of behavioural disorders, including night terrors, all types of disturbance and sexualised conduct.

This area of practice is wide ranging and generally beyond the scope of this chapter. Any professional who suspects that a child may be suffering abuse has a duty to report those suspicions to one of the statutory agencies. Social services most often take the lead, with police involvement when a criminal prosecution is contemplated or the abuse is considered relatively serious. Each NHS health trust is required to have a lead professional on child protection with whom any suspicions arising within the hospital service should be raised. Guidance on forensic examination of children suspected to have been sexually abused has been issued.[38] Further information on child sexual abuse is given in Chapter 16.

Historical allegations: the most contentious area of all?

Historical or retrospective allegations of abuse present particular difficulties for the clinician and the criminal or child protection investigation. A clinical examination is unlikely to yield diagnostic evidence but an individual may be referred with a variety of nonspecific symptoms, having made a delayed report of past abuse. In such cases, it is important that whoever investigates should examine the circumstances in which the allegation was first made and the subsequent development of the disclosures, as well as the content of the claims. While delayed claims of childhood sexual abuse may be reliable, there is always more doubt about allegations that are made long after the event, especially where there is no corroborative evidence. Time distorts the memory of events. Other peoples' views on what happened can considerably change the way that events are perceived and remembered. For all witnesses, recollection of events is altered by misunderstandings, outside pressure and sometimes intent, resulting in allegations that are unreliable.

False and mistakenly believed false allegations are now recognised to be a risk of 'therapy' where an unconscious history of childhood sexual abuse is held responsible for adult problems. In 1997, the Royal College of Psychiatrists published guidelines in the wake of concern about allegations of childhood sexual abuse made by adults in therapy.[39] The guidance advises strongly against persuasive or suggestive psychotherapeutic techniques designed to unearth sexual abuse of which the patient has no memory.

CASE E

A forensic examination was requested on a teenage girl who had been a patient in various mental health units during the past three years. Her initial admission had been for an eating disorder but now encompassed complete immobility and severe self-mutilation. At the first police involvement two years earlier, she alleged recalling memories of child sexual abuse but at that time had no idea who the perpetrator might have been. She now recounted a long history of incest with rape and buggery from a young age, which she said had been perpetrated on a daily basis over several years. She complained of generalised soreness and had not had a period for two years. Examination revealed an intact crescentic hymen, which would not admit more than the distal part of the examiner's index finger. There was no scarring or indentation and the anal findings were normal. This type of hymen is more in keeping with the non-oestrogenised prepubertal state and perhaps reflected her prolonged amenorrhoea. It also precluded the possibility that what she alleged could have taken place.

As a general rule, 'recovered memory' histories are poor indicators of specific abuse and therefore should not be relied on unless strictly corroborated. Other factors to take into account are the possibility of an underlying mental or neurological disorder and the effect of contact with other people making abuse allegations (*folie à deux*).[40]

In recent years, police investigations into historical allegations of abuse in children's homes ('trawling') have been subject to criticism as 'similar' testimony may be contaminated by the investigators and third parties.[41] Those affected may have a disturbed background including substance and alcohol abuse and a criminal record. While past abuse cannot be ruled out in these cases, such individuals may be vulnerable to confabulation and financial incentives in relation to criminal injuries compensation. An examination may, for example, be requested on a child whose parent or carer has become the subject of a historical allegation. In all these cases, it is important for the clinician to recognise that the determination of the truth or falsity of a historical uncorroborated claim may lie outside their competence and that it is therefore dangerous to interpret nonspecific findings as meaningful through being influenced by the alleged past history or psychological disturbance in the claimant of that history.[42]

Dilemmas facing medical practitioners presented with sexual assault

Where the doctor's involvement is principally in carrying out a forensic examination, they are part of the process of investigation. Their role is to help determine the facts and not to be an advocate for the complainant. Doctors are not used to this role and will have difficulty in balancing the needs of the 'patient' with their duty of impartiality.

Difficulties in the forensic service

- The management of complaints is multidisciplinary but doctors are not used to working closely with other agencies or understanding the differing needs, priorities and responsibilities of other groups:
  - ☐ forensic assessment requires an impartial open mind – open to the possibility the allegations may or may not be true.
  - ☐ therapy implies a level of advocacy for the patient.
- No reliable statistics on the true incidence and scope of sexual assault exist.
- Strong factors militate against victims making a formal complaint. Conversely, the high level of attention generated may attract some false claims.
- At present, there is wide disparity of facilities and services for examination in connection with sexual assault. In many areas, examination takes place in a police station, where there is no scope to include health related issues beyond emergency contraception.
- Victims who do complain often have important misperceptions about the forensic examination:
  - ☐ that health issues will be comprehensively covered by the examination.
  - ☐ that the examination will be able to confirm what happened.
  - ☐ that forensic samples will automatically be examined (whereas this is expensive and will only happen if there is reasonable prospect of a conviction).
- A doctor who is asked to examine an alleged victim will generally only hear one side of the story and selected facts. There is risk their interpretation of nonspecific findings may be influenced in a biased manner.

Difficulties in clinical practice

- The effects of sexual assault present to health professionals in the guise of multiple and varied symptoms which span a range of services but the diagnosis and management of sexual assault is not included in undergraduate or specialist training.
- Enquiring about sexual coercion remains a taboo that many doctors are not prepared to raise.
- Guidelines for good practice are only now being established.
- Vulnerability factors are most often determined by relationship and family dynamics.

Pitfalls for forensic medical examiners

Studies have shown that, as doctors begin their encounter with the patient, they formulate their initial hypothesis within the first minute.[43] Once an initial diagnosis is formulated, physicians tend to support their working diagnosis rather than try to refute it, so that the examination may discount findings that are not supportive.[44,45] One study has shown that doctors involved in medical examination of cases of possible sexual abuse were inconsistent in their response.[46] When given a history of possible abuse in the background information, findings, which were agreed to be natural, were put forward as strongly indicative of abuse. Findings do need to be set in context with all other information but nonspecific findings must be interpreted with extreme caution.

Conclusions

Sexual assault is traumatic when it happens but it also may have long-lasting negative effects on physical and mental health. This is a significant public health problem that has been hidden or ignored for too long. There are compelling reasons to promote the education of doctors about interpersonal violence and for its inclusion in the undergraduate curriculum. Doctors are often the first line of defence for those who cannot or are afraid to call the police. Once they look for interpersonal violence among their patients they will find it.

Although the extremes of age may be affected, the majority of sexual assault complainants are teenagers or young adults. The risk peaks among late teens, with girls aged 16–19 years being four times more likely to be assaulted or raped than the rest of the population. Most incidents occur during high-risk behaviour and most involve considerable quantities of alcohol. Vulnerability may be by age, by learning disability, or it may be due to family factors such as abusive relationships or young people with inappropriate and inconsistent boundaries.

When asked about their experience most complainants say that their treatment by the agencies could have been better.[15] In most areas forensic services are *ad hoc*, most are in police premises and offer no follow-up. Complainants are often advised to make their own arrangements with the local genitourinary medicine clinic. This does not facilitate follow-up or ensure that the health needs arising from the assault are met. Even in a well-organised woman-centred forensic service within a healthcare setting only 31% of all sexual assault victims returned for a scheduled follow-up visit.[7] Those women who do come usually have normal physical findings but may have a wide range of health-related concerns arising from their assault. At present, there is insufficient information on how best to manage these long-term health issues.

There is no legal reason that forensic examinations cannot be undertaken in various health settings, provided that collection and storage of samples observes the necessary chain of evidence. It seems likely that the most effective way to care for complainants in future will be within a setting where all health and forensic needs can be addressed. Currently, a small minority of centres meet this standard. To achieve this more widely will require a considerable increase in interagency working and a greater requirement on health trusts to provide comprehensive medical care for sexual assault.

References

1. Rape Crisis Federation Wales & England. Statistics. [www.rapecrisis.co.uk/statistics.htm].
2. US Department of Justice, Office of Justice Programs, Bureau of Justice Statistics. *Statistics from Sex offenses and Offenders. An Analysis of Data on Rape and Sexual Assault.* Washington DC; 1997. [www.ojp.usdoj.gov/bjs/abstract/soo.htm].
3. Coxell A, King M, Mezey G, Gordon D. Lifetime prevalence, characteristics and associated problems of non-consensual sex in men: cross sectional survey. *BMJ* 1999;318:846–50.
4. MacDonald R. Time to talk about rape. *BMJ* 2000;321:1034–5.
5. Home Office. Recorded Crime Statistics 1898–2001/02. [www.homeoffice.gov.uk/rds/pdfs/100years.xls].
6. Cloutier S, Martin SL, Poole C. Sexual assault among North Carolina women: Prevalence and Health risk factors. *J Epidemiol Community Health* 2002;56:265–71.
7. Holmes MM, Resnick HS, Frampton D. Follow-up of sexual assault victims. *Am J Obstet Gynecol* 1998;179:336–42.
8. Ritchie EC. Reactions to rape: a military forensic psychiatrists perspective. *Mil Med* 1998;163:505–9.
9. McFarlane AC, DeGirolamo G. The nature of traumatic stressors and the epidemiology of posttraumatic reactions. In: van der Kolk BA, McFarlane AC, Weisaeth L, editors. *Traumatic Stress: The Effects of Overwhelming Experience on Mind, Body and Society.* New York: Guilford Press; 1996. p. 241–56.
10. American Psychiatric Association. *Diagnostic and Statistical Manual of Mental Disorders DSM-IV.* Arlington, VA: American Psychiatric Press; 1994.
11. Kenardy J. The current status of psychological debriefing: it may do more harm than good. *BMJ* 2000;321:1032–3.
12. Herman JL. *Trauma and Recovery. The Aftermath of Violence: From Domestic Abuse to Political Terror.* 2nd ed. London: Rivers Oram/Pandora; 2001.
13. Personal View. The day my life changed. *BMJ* 2000;321:1089.
14. Home Office Woman's Unit. *Living Without Fear: An Integrated Approach to Tackling Violence Against Women.* London: Home Office; 1999.
15. Sturman P. *Drug Assisted Sexual Assault: A Study for the Home Office Under the Police Research Award Scheme.* London: Home Office; 2001. [http://www.shirepro.co.uk/drugrape.pdf].
16. Sexual assault in adults. *Drug Ther Bull* 2002;40:1–4.
17. Riggs N, Houry D, Long G, Markovchick V, Feldhaus KM. Analysis of 1,076 cases of sexual assault. *Ann Emerg Med* 2000;35:358–62.
18. Tyra PA. Older women: Victims of rape. *J Gerontol Nurs* 1993;19:7–12.
19. Ramrakha S, Caspi A, Dickson N, Moffitt TE, Paul C. Psychiatric disorders and risky sexual behaviour in young adulthood: cross sectional study in birth cohort. *BMJ* 2000;321:263–6.
20. Dickson N, Paul C, Herbison P, Silva P. First sexual intercourse: age, coercion and later regrets reported by a birth cohort. *BMJ* 1998;316:29–33.
21. Koss MP. Hidden rape: sexual aggression and victimization in the national sample of students in higher education. In: Pirog-Good MA, Stets JE, editors. *Violence in Dating Relationships: Emerging Social Issues.* New York: Praeger; 1988. p. 145–68.
22. Warshaw R. *I Never Called It Rape.* New York: HarperPerennial; 1994.
23. Koss MP, Dinero TE. A discriminant analysis of risk factors among a national sample of college women. *J Consult Clin Psychol* 1988;57:133–47.
24. Hendessi M. *Voices of Children Witnessing Domestic Violence: A Form of Child Abuse.* Coventry: Coventry Domestic Violence Focus Group; 1997.
25. Campbell JC. Health consequences of intimate partner violence. *Lancet* 2002;359:1331–6.

26. Williamson E. *Domestic Violence and Health: The Response of the Medical Profession*. Bristol: Policy Press 2000.

27. Long FY, Pang E, Kee C. Pilot study to assess the viability of a rape trauma syndrome questionnaire. *Ann Acad Med Singapore* 2002;31:777–84.

28. Kirk-Weir I. Evaluating child sexual abuse. *Family Law* 1996;673–7.

29. Meadow R. Dilemmas. In: Meadow R, editor. *ABC of Child Abuse*. 3rd ed. London: BMJ Publishing Group. p. 51–3.

30. Pillai M. Allegations of Abuse: the need for responsible practice. *Med Sci Law* 2002;42:149–59.

31. Bowyer L, Dalton ME. Female victims of rape and their genital injuries. *Br J Obstet Gynaecol* 1997;104:617–20.

32. Miller G, Stermac L, Addison M. Immediate and delayed treatment seeking among adult sexual assault victims. *Women and Health* 2002;35:53–64.

33. Association of Genito Urinary Medicine and Medical Society for the Study of Venereal Diseases. Clinical Effectiveness Group. *National Guidelines on the Management of Adult Victims of Sexual Assault*. Nottingham; 2001.

34. Estreich S, Forster GE, Robinson A. Sexually transmitted diseases in rape victims. *Genitourin Med* 1990;66:433–6.

35. Jenny C, Hooton TM, Bowers A, Copass MK, Krieger JN, Hillier SL, *et al.* STDs in victims of rape. *N Engl J Med* 1990;322:713–16.

36. Dalton VK, Haefner HK, Reed BD, Senapati S, Cook A. Victimisation in patients with vulvar dysesthesia/vestibulodynia. Is there and increased prevalence? *J Reprod Med* 2002;47:829–34.

37. Norton LB, Peipert JF, Zierler S, Lima B, Hume L. Battering in pregnancy: an assessment of two screening methods. *Obstet Gynaecol* 1995;85:321–5.

38. Royal College of Paediatrics and Child Health, Association of Police Surgeons. *Guidance on Paediatric Forensic Examinations in Relation to Possible Child Sexual Abuse*. London; 2002.

39. Royal College of Psychiatrists Reported recovered memories of child sexual abuse: recommendations for good practice and implications for training, continuing professional development and research. *Psychiatric Bull* 1997;21:663–5.

40. Boakes J. False complaints of sexual assault: recovered memories of childhood sexual abuse. *Med Sci Law* 1998;39:112–20.

41. Webster R. *The Great Children's Home Panic*. Oxford: Orwell Press; 1998.

42. Piper A, Pope HG, Borowiecki JF. Custer's last stand: Brown Scheflin and Whitfield's latest attempt to salvage "dissociative amnesia" *J Psychiatr Law* 2000;28,149–213.

43. Barrows HS, Norman GR, Neufeld VR, Feightner JW. The clinical reasoning of randomly selected physicians in general medical practice. *Clin Invest Med* 1982;5:49–55.

44. Muram D, Arheart KL, Jennings SG. The diagnostic accuracy of colposcopic photographs in child sexual abuse evaluations. *J Pediatr Adolesc Gynecol* 1999;12:58–61.

45. Muram D. The medical evaluation in cases of child sexual abuse. *J Pediatr Adolesc Gynecol* 1999;14:55–64.

46. Roberts REI. Forensic medical evidence in rape and child sexual abuse: controversies and a possible solution. *J R Soc Med* 1999;92:388–92.

Chapter 4

Consent

Michael Wilks and Maureen Dalton

Introduction

Clearly, in most, if not all cases of alleged sexual assault, a major issue to be determined by the courts will be that of consent by the alleged victim to sexual intercourse. Therefore, the capacity of that person and whether capacity was, at the time of the alleged offence, undermined by illness, either physical or mental, or by alcohol or drugs, may well be something upon which the medical examiner will be asked to provide an opinion in evidence. Observations on these matters should therefore be a matter of careful note keeping.

This chapter, however, is concerned with the issue of consent by the victim to medical examination, to the collection of forensic samples and the disclosure of medical evidence in the form of documents to be presented to court. That said, the issue of consent to intercourse and consent to examination and disclosure will, in many cases, be linked. If a victim is unable, for a variety of possible reasons, to give fully informed consent to examination soon after an assault, it follows that her capacity to consent to intercourse may have equally been impaired. These are linked factors that the doctor may be asked to consider in oral or written evidence.

One of the four great principles of medical ethics, autonomy (literally 'self rule') is central to the issue of consent. The 'gold standard' of consent to medical treatment is that of a fully informed patient, with full capacity, being able to make autonomous judgements about what the doctor is proposing to undertake. It has often been argued that this is an impossible ideal to achieve. All patients have different levels of need, understanding, knowledge and insight. It is the doctor's responsibility to provide the right amount of information relevant to that particular patient's needs at that particular time. This is, to say the least, difficult and requires an initial assessment of the patient's needs and capacity.

Capacity to consent can be diminished or varied by illness, mental incapacity, intoxication or age. It must be debatable whether a victim of a recent assault has that capacity, particularly in relation to the disclosure of information, much of which is highly sensitive and personal, at the time of examination. Arguably, there are different balances of harm and benefit when it comes to examination. The benefits of conducting early examination and sampling in the interests of the investigation of a criminal act demand that the doctor should attempt to overcome initial reluctance to examination and proceed on an assumption of implied consent. Obviously, where there is refusal, the doctor cannot proceed but can still make observations and record findings for which consent to disclosure can be sought at a later date.

When it comes to disclosure itself, different principles apply. It is unlikely that a traumatised victim of a recent assault has the capacity to think through the consequences of a disclosure of past sexual or reproductive history when it comes to cross-examination in court. This is a matter that will usually need to be discussed at a later stage, when the immediate trauma is past. In many cases, this will be a necessary step, as the victim may well be suspected of being under the influence of alcohol or drugs at the time of the assault and/or examination.

It follows from this that:

■ consent for examination and sampling will usually be adequate to allow the doctor to proceed, in the interests of collecting evidence
■ consent for disclosure will usually be absent and will need to be obtained at a later date.

Consent for examination

As has been stated, respect for patient autonomy requires that a doctor can only proceed with examination and investigation if the patient has capacity (or competence) and knowledge (or information). Capacity has to be assessed and knowledge has to be provided. The assessment of capacity[1] is a complex process and, essentially, requires a judgement to made as to whether the patient possesses the characteristics of insight and self determination, that is the ability to process information, consider its relevance to current circumstances and then make a valid decision. In the majority of adult victims, there will be sufficient capacity to proceed with necessary examination and investigations, even if the patient's capacity is temporarily impaired by distress or by alcohol and/or drugs. This is so because there is usually, if not always, a benefit to proceeding. The benefit will almost always be present in the case of the patient, as thorough investigation of an assault can rarely said to be against their interest. In addition, however, benefit will always be present in the interests of justice, as the competent and thorough collection of evidence will assist in creating a correct balance between the interests of victim and assailant. It must be remembered that the forensic examiner, as a truly independent agent, has a wider responsibility than the examination of the patient. Information obtained from that examination may be disclosed, in full, at the direction of the court and may well serve to protect the interests of those falsely accused of a major offence.

There will, however, be circumstances in which the victim will be so distressed or so impaired that informed consent cannot be obtained. How the doctor proceeds in such cases must be a matter of individual judgement, depending on the urgency of obtaining evidence and the anticipated period of time before sufficient capacity is restored. When doctors are asked to examine alleged victims who are unconscious and, therefore, under the care of a hospital, again, a balance of harm and benefit must be reached. Good practice in these circumstances requires:

- that the consultant responsible for the medical care of the patient is informed as to the nature and purpose of the proposed examination to ensure that there is no objection to it being undertaken
- that any close 'family' members or carers able to be contacted are alerted to the nature and purpose of the proposed examination, in order to determine whether the patient had made them aware of any previously relevant views (it should be noted that, in the case of an adult patient, a family member is not able to consent or refuse on their behalf)
- whenever possible, that a family member or carer who knows the patient is present during the examination
- that all steps in this process are fully documented
- that, in the event of the patient's recovery, she is informed as to what has been done and retrospective consent obtained.[2]

In general, the provision of information in an accessible way is vital if the goal of fully informed consent is to be achieved. Many doctors fall back on familiar terms when explaining to their patients what they propose to do and why. These terms may well be familiar to them, but unfamiliar to their patients. What is required in the forensic examination of a victim of sexual assault is, clearly, empathy and time, but also a clear initial explanation of the doctor's role. Being a doctor should immediately raise an understanding of an essentially caring and therapeutic role but it is important also to explain the 'dual responsibility' that the doctor has. There is a primary duty of confidence and care but this is qualified by the responsibility to act not necessarily in the interests of the police but of the judicial process. This is extremely difficult to put across to a young woman whose plans for the evening did not include spending time in a victim examination suite and for whom the whole experience is traumatic and unfamiliar. Simple and repeated explanation will be needed and time given to allow understanding to develop and for questions to be asked. Only when this process is complete is there likely to be sufficient consent for examination.

A related issue will be consent for treatment. There will usually be issues around screening for genitourinary infections and pregnancy. These will involve taking consent for referral to an appropriate specialist clinic or a general practitioner. Again, consent for this, being normally in the patient's best interest, should be sought at this time.

The victim has a right to confidentiality and secrecy. She may well have brought a friend or member of her family with her to support her but it should not be assumed that she is happy to have them present at all times. The same principle applies to any police officers present.

Consent to disclosure

Disclosure of forensic medical records is covered by the general principles relating to third-party disclosure. These are that medical information about a patient can only be provided to another party with that patient's fully informed consent. This must include an understanding of:

- what information is required
- why it is needed
- to whom it will be disclosed.

The General Medical Council (GMC) states that "patients have a right to expect that you will not disclose information which you learnt during the course of your professional duties, unless they give permission".[3] Circumstances in which consent for disclosure can be ignored are uncommon and have, according to the GMC, to be justified on the grounds of "serious risk to others".[3] The GMC makes it clear that the investigation of a crime and the provision to a third party, such as investigating officer, are not in themselves sufficient to satisfy the test of "serious" risk.[3] Such disclosures require consent, and good practice therefore requires, in many cases, a different standard to that applying to consent for examination. This is because there is a different balance of interest. In relation to consent for examination, as has been stated, there is a combination of, sometimes conflicting, personal and general interests. In the case of disclosure, the balance is firmly on the side of the patient's (often highly) personal interest, because the information collected by the doctor may have no relevance to the case and its disclosure may be both unnecessary and harmful.

At this point, two important points must be made. First, that the doctor has limited knowledge of the facts of the case and can therefore not be in a position to judge what is relevant information and what is not. Some (particularly defence lawyers) would therefore argue that full disclosure at an early stage is the only way to ensure that all relevant factors are considered. Others would argue that what is required is an early disclosure of what is relevant, based on an assessment of the main evidential strands in the case as soon as possible but not immediately after the assault. The second point is that medical information has no absolute confidence. It can be divulged in court, at the court's direction. The doctor can argue, in the interests of the patient, that certain facts are irrelevant to the case. Such arguments can be heard in private session. However, the final decision on the relevance of any information recorded by the doctor is a matter for the court.

The prosecution has an obligation to identify evidential material that, even if not forming part of the prosecution case, must be disclosed to the defence.[4] In R v Keane,[5] Lord Taylor of Gosforth stated: "The prosecution must identify the documents and information which are material ... Having identified what is material, the prosecution should disclose it unless they wish to maintain that public interest immunity or other sensitivity justifies withholding some or all of it".

It therefore follows that good practice must recognise these often conflicting principles. Consent to disclosure should be taken only when the patient has the capacity and the information to make an informed decision. In the case of an examination some time after an event, these factors are likely to be present. In the case of a recent assault, they may be, but the doctor may still consider it wise that they should be revisited at a later date. The question then arises as to the responsibility of the doctor, as opposed to others concerned in the investigation, to undertake this task. In many cases it will be impracticable for the doctor to have a further meeting with the victim. The Association of Police Surgeons and the Crown Prosecution Service are agreed that it is not in the interests of justice that important medical evidence is made available at a late stage in the preparation of a case and that, therefore, a mechanism should exist to allow this to be disclosed as early as is practicable. Late disclosure of essential information can lead to a great deal of unnecessary work preparing a case that would not be taken to court if earlier disclosure had been made. Equally, it may be in the interests of a victim either to know that this is the case. The Association of Police Surgeons and the Crown Prosecution Service are jointly preparing an information sheet for victims of sexual assault in relation to disclosure of medical evidence.[6] This can be given to the victim in advance of a later approach for informed consent. While it may be helpful for this second approach to involve a doctor, it could be delegated to an officer who will, after all, have experience in understanding victims' needs.

Current guidance, produced jointly by the Association of Police Surgeons and the Royal College of Paediatrics and Child Health includes advice in relation to photography.[7] It is increasingly common for forensic examiners to take photographs. These form part of the medical record and are treated in terms of disclosure in the same way as any other documents. Consent for their taking and use should be included in the routine processes relating to examination and disclosure. Photographs are also useful teaching aids. Consent in relation to examination covers their use in the interests of the patient's medical care but not for teaching purposes. Separate, informed consent, usually at a later stage, will be required for this purpose. However, there has to be an acknowledgement about the sensitive nature of these photographs and who has access to them. The Newcastle and Durham Judiciary have recently produced a guideline for the handling of these sensitive images, confirming that they are only to be viewed by medical experts unless a judge directs otherwise. This allows the woman the confidence to consent to colpodocumentation if it is considered appropriate. This guideline is included here as Appendix 4.1.

References

1.   British Medical Association, Law Society. *Assessment of Mental Capacity: Guidance for Doctors and Lawyers*. 2nd ed. London: BMJ Books; 2004.
2.   British Medical Association, Medical Ethics Department. Card 5: Assessment of competence. Consent tool kit. 2nd ed. February 2003. [www.bma.org.uk/ap.nsf/Content/consenttk2%5C5].
3.   General Medical Council. Seeking patients' consent: the ethical considerations. November 1998 [www.gmc-uk.org/standards/default.htm].
4.   Crown Prosecution Service. Legal Guidance. Disclosure and Covert Law Enforcement. Disclosure of unused material [www.cps.gov.uk/Home/LegalGuidance/20/20-F.pdf].
5.   R v Keane (1994) 99 Cr. App.R1.
6.   Association of Forensic Physicians, Royal College of Paediatrics and Child Health. Information sheet for victims of sexual assault in relation to disclosure of medical evidence. [www.apsweb.org.uk/text/publications.shtml GUIDELINES/ADVICE]
7.   Association of Forensic Physicians, Royal College of Paediatrics and Child Health. guidance in relation to photography. [www.apsweb.org.uk/text/publications.shtml GUIDELINES/ADVICE]

Appendix 4.1
A protocol for the management of highly sensitive images in the criminal justice system

In the Crown Courts at Newcastle upon Tyne and Durham

1. This protocol shall apply to the management of highly sensitive images within the criminal justice system in the Northumbria Police and Durham Police areas.

Objectives

2. The object of the protocol is to ensure respect for the privacy of the subjects of the highly sensitive images and to eliminate the risk of improper distribution of the highly sensitive images.

Definitions

3. A highly sensitive image is a photographic or video image of the genitalia or anus of a child, young person or adult, of either sex and the breasts of a female child, young person or adult, which comes into being during the course of an investigation into suspected sexual or physical abuse of the subject of the image.
4. A judge of the Crown Court is a High Court Judge, a Circuit Judge and a Recorder who is permitted to try serious sexual offences.

Medical examiners

5. A medical examiner shall state in any report or witness statement whether a photographic or video image has or has not been made during a medical examination into suspected sexual or physical abuse.

Management of highly sensitive images

6. This original of a highly sensitive image shall be retained as part of the subject's medical records.
7. A copy of a highly sensitive image shall be provided on request only to medical experts instructed in the case and only on the giving of the undertakings set out in Appendix 1 by that expert, which includes an

undertaking not to show the highly sensitive image to any person, save another medical expert, without the permission of a Judge of the Crown Court.

8. Applications for a copy of a highly sensitive image or for sight of the original or an existing copy, by a person who is not a medical expert, shall be made to a Judge of the Crown Court, preferably at the plea and directions hearing.

9. Applications under paragraph 8 shall not be granted unless:
   i) the Judge has heard representations made by or on behalf of the medical examiner who holds the original and
   ii) the Judge is satisfied that the interests of justice so demand and shall only be granted on such terms, including the giving of undertakings, which ensure, so far as is possible, the objectives of this Protocol set out at paragraph 2.

10. At the conclusion of the case all copies of a highly sensitive image must be returned to the medical examiner who made the original image. Receipt thereof must be acknowledged by the medical examiner and the copies must be destroyed, unless consent has been given, by or on behalf of the subject of the highly sensitive image, for the same to be retained for medical teaching purposes or peer review.

Marking

11. A copy of a highly sensitive image is to be contained within a covering which clearly marks that within the covering there is a highly sensitive image.

12. If a brief to counsel or a higher court advocate contains a copy of a highly sensitive image, that fact should be clearly marked on the backsheet.

His Honour Judge Hodson
The Honorary Recorder of Newcastle upon Tyne

His Honour Judge Lowden
Resident Judge at Durham Crown Court

Dated March 2003

Appendix 1

Undertaking to be given and signed by any person who takes possession of a highly sensitive image.

I undertake that whilst the highly sensitive image in the case of R v _____ _____ is in my possession I shall:

a) not permit any other person, save another medical expert, to see the highly sensitive image without permission of the Court

b) not cause or permit any copy to be made of the highly sensitive image

c) record the name and address of any medical expert to whom I have shown the highly sensitive image

d) ensure that the highly sensitive image is always kept in a locked, secure container, save when in use, and not left in an unattended vehicle or otherwise left unprotected

e) return the highly sensitive image by a secure route to the medical examiner who holds the original, at the conclusion of the case or when I am no longer professionally involved in the case.

Chapter 5

Taking a history

Hazel Walter and Maureen Dalton

Introduction

The doctor who wears both a forensic and a medical, caring hat in the forensic medical assessment should be able to facilitate the start of the therapeutic recovery, so that the assessment is not another ordeal for the complainant. It is primarily the police officer's responsibility to obtain a detailed investigative history. The police have an important role in the complainant's experience and decision to continue with the case. The examining doctor must, however, take a precise and accurate history of the incident to ensure that an appropriate examination is undertaken and the collection of forensic evidence is complete. A forensic medical examiner assisting the court during a trial needs to be able to demonstrate that they have been thorough and impartial in carrying out the assessment of a sexual assault complainant and have drawn proper conclusions in the light of the information gleaned from the forensic medical assessment.

The practice of using protocols for forensic medical examinations is becoming accepted and locally devised pro forma assessment sheets with clear checklists for the historical facts and for the examination may assist the examiner in gaining the necessary information to treat any possible injuries and to adapt the standardised gynaecological forensic examination according to the circumstances. The Association of Forensic Physicians (formerly the Association of Police Surgeons) has an example of such a pro forma, which is included here as Appendix 5.1. Personal notes should be taken in such a way that they can be read by others and easily identifiable (signed with the full name in printed form).

Initial contact by police

When first telephoned, the forensic medical examiner may be given some details of the assault and may need to give advice over the telephone. This might include recommendations about the bagging of clothes, including what to do about large, very wet or heavily bloodstained items, the taking of urine or oral samples and the collection of a sanitary towel or tampon, if it is being changed prior to the examination.

Procedure at the examination suite

Explaining the role of the forensic medical examiner

Prior to the arrival of the forensic medical examiner, the police officer should have shown the complainant around the examination centre and explained the roles of the personnel involved in her care. One of the principal aims of those involved in forensic examination of sexual assault complainants should be to minimise the mental and physical trauma to the woman while endeavouring to collect useful forensic evidence in as dignified and understanding manner as possible. When first walking into the room, the examiner should quickly make good eye contact with the complainant. The complainant will be feeling scared and worthless and if she also feels that the examiner is only talking to the policewoman it will reinforce these feelings. Following the usual introductions, the forensic medical examiner should explain the purpose of the examination, gaining written consent prior to checking her medical needs and subsequent medical and forensic examination plus collection of forensic samples. Other consent issues can be covered as they arise.

Discussion between the police officer and the forensic medical examiner

Prior to the doctor engaging with the complainant, the police officer will usually provide the forensic medical examiner with a summary of the events and the allegation.

Personnel details

It is important to ensure that contact details are sought from each individual present, including those with whom telephone contact has previously been made and the trained police officer present, officers or doctors in training, the investigation officers (CID) and, where applicable, the interpreter and the social worker.

It is important to enquire about and document the contact point for a completed statement. Details of family members or friends present are recorded. Details of the complainant's general practitioner and any counsellor, psychologist or psychiatrist are also recorded, to allow details of events to be forwarded if the complainant so wishes.

Relevant medical, psychiatric and social history

Consent must be gained for the medical history, the examination, the taking of samples, the use of photography or colposcopic examination, and the use of anonymised data for other doctors, which entails having some background information from the individual early on in the process. The complainant's ability to consent may be assessed while listening to the individual describing her health concerns, occupational details, educational achievements or hobbies (see Chapter 4).

By obtaining a medical and social history early on in the proceedings, the examiner aims to put the complainant at ease rather than escalating her distress by obtaining an account of the events that precipitated her referral.

A helpful way of explaining about the collection of medical details is to say that the court needs to consider the cause of any mark or injury, which is difficult if you do not know the background health of the patient.

The forensic medical examiner may continue to give examples of details required to assess skin findings, such as any bruising tendency or known skin conditions, and to emphasise how important it is to know about drugs prescribed or not prescribed, together with any over-the-counter preparations and substance use and abuse. Details about current medical concerns or disabilities should be recorded, together with relevant past medical and surgical information and relevant obstetric and gynaecological history, which should include details about childbirth, surgery and current contraception.

Particular attention should be paid to certain aspects of information of the patient's background and, in particular, to any addictive disorders and certain mental health problems. There is also a need to be aware of the up-to-date terminology for different sexual activities, street drugs and commonly used alcohol-containing drinks.

Useful questions may include: " Do you have any problems with your chest or tummy or waterworks?". Varying the vocabulary according to the patient's own terms for body parts and functions while trying to avoid leading them may also prove useful.

Details about sexual activity

It is important to find out whether the complainant has ever had sexual intercourse and, if so, to record the date of intercourse occurring within the past 14 days and with whom. For such intercourse, the forensic medical examiner needs to record whether a condom, spermicide or other lubricant or contraceptive was used.

History of the event

It is important to be sensitive to the patient's needs yet to obtain information that will help those investigating the allegation, including the forensic science laboratory, the Crown Prosecution Service and the court. The standard pro forma is very detailed but remember it is simply an aid to memory.

The source of each piece of information should be documented. Initially, the details are taken down verbatim. Unless the officer has suggested otherwise, this should be done in front of the complainant. On completion of the officer's knowledge of events, the complainant should be asked if the details are accurate and if she wishes to add anything.

The date and time of the incident, together with the time lapse, are important details to document. A history of the place of assault and types of surface on which it occurred may help with the later interpretation of marks or injuries.

It is important to establish whether or not the complainant felt that a weapon or implement was used at the incident or whether there was damage to her clothing. If she indicates she has been injured, she should be asked about the site of the injuries and how she perceives they were sustained. Should an injury or mark be identified later on, during the examination (see Chapter 6), which has not been alluded to in the history taking, it is then necessary to ask how and when it occurred, without giving any suggestions as to causation. The details of this later conversation should be recorded, indicating that these facts were obtained after the original history taking.

It may be useful for the police if, early on in the investigation, information about lost articles, including clothing, condoms, tissues, make-up, jewellery and bags, can be obtained, as they may be searching a sealed-off site. The accompanying officer may be able to contact the police at the scene immediately to alert their attention to the missing articles.

Events following the incident

A brief history of events following the incident should be taken, together with full details of the complainant's subsequent cleansing. It is important to establish whether she has had further sexual activity since the incident and to detail it, also including details of food, drink and drugs or medication taken.

Dilemmas

Reliability of information

The complainant may come into contact with and provide details of her assault to several professionals involved in her care. The extent to which the forensic medical examiner should go to establish the source of each component of her history not personally given is not clear. For example, in this chain of involvement, the first person to be provided with details of the incident may be an officer in the police station or control room, who then passes the information to a trained officer in sexual assault investigation.

Whether or not the forensic medical examiner should record all the details of each officer's name, rank, identification number and contact number and from whom they obtained their version of events is debatable. The court considers 'first complaint' details to be important.

The person accompanying the complainant may be able to provide fuller details, which should be noted, as they may differ from those given by the complainant. This difference may cause confusion for the investigating officers; indeed, it may be used in court to attempt to show lack of thoroughness on the part of the forensic medical examiner. Differing recollections of what happened is common and does not make the allegation invalid.

History of the incident

Taking the medical history in the traditional way will provide a lot of details about which some doctors are unhappy, as they feel that this is intrusive, unnecessary and may be contentious in court. Assessing what is relevant, pertinent, or recent is often debated but comes with experience.

Details of the assailant or assailants

How far the forensic medical examiner should go in obtaining information about the assailant or assailants is unclear. Details volunteered by the complainant should be recorded and could assist in the early arrest of the assailant, particularly in a 'stranger' rape. The details may reveal a *modus operandi* that is already known to other police forces and may be useful to track down serial rapists. Those working on intelligence data of serial rapists and murderers have details of assailants on computer databases and assault details requested in the following pro forma have been prompted by their work (see Appendix 5.1).

Direct questioning

Even if the forensic medical examiner is objective, non-judgemental and sensitive to the woman's needs, it can be extremely difficult and time consuming to obtain details of the incident. One must not assume that a bizarre disclosure means that the allegation is false. Despite the temptation to do otherwise, only indirect open-ended questions should be used to ascertain the assault history. If it appears that the history is one of vagino-penile penetration only, it is important to give the complainant plenty of opportunity to disclose that other forms of sexual activity occurred even though they may feel highly embarrassed or ashamed of them. It can be difficult to address such issues without direct questioning. Suggested open-ended questions include:

- Did anything else happen to you?
- Were you made to do anything?
- Did any other activity occur in different parts of your body?
- Were you touched anywhere else?

Frequently, at the beginning of the consultation, the complainant may feel that the story is all too awful to tell. It may be that, later, during the examination, prompts can be used again. The information may come spontaneously at the time of genital examination. Never assume that no disclosure means that nothing has happened.

Changes in the complainant's allegation

If the complainant adds new details, these must be recorded verbatim. These changes in the account written in the doctor's personal notes may be requested by the court later. It may be that, when the complainant has calmed down, she may remember more clearly the exact details of what happened. In court, the counsel for the defence may make much of the variation in the complainant's account and try to make it appear that the complainant had fabricated the incident.

Changes in the story may be just due to the fact that the receiver of the story did not use the verbatim words but used their own interpretation. It is vitally important therefore to be accurate at all times.

Having no clear recollection of events does not necessarily mean that it is a false allegation. It may be an indication of substance-mediated assault. In the UK, at present, forensic science laboratories are finding a high level of alcohol is the most common substance on toxicological assessment and other substances much less frequently.

Pro forma prompts

The nature of the pro forma suggests that there should be complete details about the assault. However, if the information requested in the pro forma is not revealed in the account given then it is important to leave the prompt spaces blank. The forensic medical examiner must not ask direct questions as it may encourage the suggestible witness to enlarge the story in order to be believed.

Use of colloquial terms

It can be difficult for the forensic medical examiner to appreciate the latest street terms for alcohol or other substances. Care needs to be taken with the details recorded otherwise the examiner may be misled when assessing the complainant for intoxication of these substances. Throughout, the forensic medical examiner should use lay terminology.

Sensitivity to the difficulties of interpreters and signers

Interpreters may have little training and support in the field of sexual abuse and rape, especially in relation to younger complainants. This can sometimes be difficult when they find the words used by the complainant upsetting and difficult to translate, especially if pet or family-specific words are used for parts of the genital anatomy. Their own life experiences may not have prepared them for what they have heard. The interpreter may also disapprove of the former lifestyle of the complainant. The examiner needs to be sensitive to this problem and be aware that the interpretation of colloquial words may be quite misleading.

Bizarre allegations

It is important to take the complaint at face value. First hearing may provide some incredible stories. It is considered that false complaints are not common. The forensic medical examiner should bear in mind that the very young, those with learning difficulties and elderly women may not understand what rape is or know the terminology to describe the assault. Adolescents may not give an exact story, as they may be protecting someone or may be making a complaint for other short-term gain, especially those who exhibit considerable disturbed behaviour. It is in this age group that false or partly false allegations occur most often.

The initial disclosure may come falsely from an adult about a young person who is concerned for the complainant's welfare or has been angered by their apparently irresponsible behaviour.

It is rare to discontinue an examination because the false allegation is clear. Occasionally, the patient may be frankly psychotic with delusions (describing acts of penetration from 60 feet, for example). It must not be forgotten, however, that people with mental health problems may be particularly vulnerable to sexual assault. To consider an allegation false there must be clear firm evidence rather than a suspicion. Even admissions of false allegation by the patient may prove later to be incorrect but are offered because of fear of reprisal.

Medical history: brevity, detail and relevance

Our medical training leads us to become accustomed to seeking as much background information about our patients, including their social, educational and general medical details, using direct questions for speed. This completeness may provide a dilemma to the physician, who tends to be wary of the court system, with a perceived need to protect 'their' patient by being thrifty with details. This may make the forensic medical examiner appear to be biased and partisan in court, thus undermining the credibility of the forensic medical examiner as a professional witness.

The minimalist view is to leave out specific details, which may be taken to be contentious in court, but how do doctors know what will be contentious in court? Examples of medical and social details that are often excluded or avoided include:

- terminations of pregnancy
- treatment for sexually transmitted infections
- divorce proceedings
- children in care
- addictive disorder
- psychiatric illness
- previous suicide attempts
- child abuse
- self harm.

It is important to include in the statement a reference to the fact that the conclusions are based on the information given at the time of the examination and that if further relevant information emerges the conclusions may require modification. Also remember that it is part of the role of the good defence barrister to try to find fault with your conduct of the case in the hope that they can convince the jury that your evidence is not worth considering. They may therefore often pick holes in your history.

Particulars about previous counselling, psychological help of any sort and past psychiatric diagnoses and treatment may be important to the forensic medical examiner's advice and action on follow-up plans for safety. Advice to the police about a vulnerable patient's anxieties concerning safety and immediate mental health care may be important. It may be necessary to prompt the investigating officer to ask a named consultant in mental health to give advice to the court about the patient's problems (with consent). Details of self-harming and overdose attempts may be relevant.

With respect to psychiatric illness, it may be in the best interests of the complainant to disclose full details to the court, to allow professionals involved in the care of the complainant to provide additional and possibly supportive details of relevance to the proceedings. If the psychiatric background is withheld and later it is revealed that the complainant has a psychopathy that has led to a false complaint the forensic medical examiner may end up being discredited for wasting the court's time.

Details about which the patient is unclear may suggest a need to gain information from the general practitioner or the relevant hospital consultant (with consent) before interpretation and conclusion formulation in the statement.

Who should be present during the history taking and examination?

On the whole, the complainant should feel that she is in control and decide for herself who should accompany her during the interview and examination. There may be occasions when the forensic medical examiner has to intervene. For example:

- A man accompanying an adolescent was asked by the adolescent to stay throughout the whole procedure. He claimed that he had been sent in place of her mother, with whom he was cohabiting, The man had no actual legal right to expect to be involved. He was firmly but sensitively advised that it was inappropriate for him to be present during the procedure. Much later on it was discovered that he had been sexually abusing the adolescent.
- A boyfriend who was intoxicated with alcohol (as was the patient) was obstructive and disinhibited when he insisted on being present. It took some time to encourage him to leave the consulting room.
- A trained police officer may insist on being present. Should the complainant indicate that she does not wish the officer to be present, the forensic medical examiner should try to reach a compromise that leaves the complainant feeling in control. For example, the officer could be asked to stay on the other side of the screen or curtain until the clothes are handed over for bagging and then to leave the room to seal the bagged items. The complainant may then agree to the officer coming back into the room at the end of the examination to assist the forensic medical examiner in the labelling and sealing of exhibits. For practical purposes, it is much easier and quicker to have the discreet assistance of the officer who also acts as a chaperone for the examiner.

Access to the forensic medical examiner's record of the examination

Counsel for the defence may request the contemporaneous notes. It is probably wise practice to confirm again with the complainant that she is still prepared for her details to be released. Consideration should be given to obtaining further consent for disclosure. If consent for the personal notes to be shown in court is obtained at the initial examination, before the investigation is complete, it could be said that the consent was not fully informed.

The General Medical Council[1-3] and joint Association of Police Surgeons and British Medical Association[4] guidelines on confidentiality and consent may be consulted.

If there are any concerns about withholding information after a judge's order, seek legal advice for this, either from the NHS trust lawyers or personal insurance legal advisers, in order not to fall foul of a contempt of court ruling or the General Medical Council's confidentiality code.

References

1. General Medical Council. *Confidentiality*. London; September 2000 [www.gmc-uk.org/standards/default.htm].
2. General Medical Council. *Good Medical Practice*. 3rd ed. London; May 2001 [www.gmc-uk.org/standards/default.htm].
3. General Medical Council. *Seeking Patients' Consent: The Ethical Considerations*. London; November 1998 [www.gmc-uk.org/standards/default.htm].
4. Association of Police Surgeons, British Medical Association. *Revised Interim Guidelines on Confidentiality for Police Surgeons in England, Wales and Northern Ireland*. February 1998. Available from: Medical Ethics Departments, BMA House, Tavistock Square, London WC1H 9JP; telephone +44 (0) 171 383 6286; fax +44 (0) 171 383 6233; or the Association of Forensic Physicians, Penvern, Nacton, Ipswich IP10 0EW; telephone +44 (0) 1473 659014 [www.afpweb.org.uk/files/confidentiality.doc].

Additional reading

Bezchlibnyk-Butler KZ, Jeffries JJ. *Clinical Handbook of Psychotropic Drugs*. Toronto: Hogrefe & Huber; 1996.

Cowen PJ, Nutt DJ. Abstinence syndromes after withdrawal of tranquillising drugs. *Lancet* 1982;ii:360–2.

Crowley RC. *Sexual Assault: The Medico-legal Examination*. Stamford, CT: Appleton & Lange; 1999.

General Medical Council. *Intimate Examinations*. London; December 2001 [www.gmc-uk.org/standards/default.htm].

Goodwin J, Sahd D, Rada R. *False Accusations and False Denials of Incest: Clinical Myths and Clinical Realities*. In: Goodwin J, editor. *Sexual Abuse, Incest Victims, and Their Families*. Boston: John Wright; 1982. p.17–26.

Greenfield L. *An Analysis of Data on Rape and Sexual Assault: Sex Offenses and Offenders* (NCJ-163392). Washington DC: Bureau of Justice Statistics, US Department of Justice; 1997.

Karch SB. Dermatological sequelae of opiate abuse. In: Karch SB. *The Pathology of Drug Abuse*. 2nd ed. Boca Raton, FL: CRC Press; 1996. p. 348–54.

Macdowell C, Hibler N. False allegations. In: Hazelwood R, Burgess AW, editors. *Practical Aspects of Rape Investigation: A Multi-Disciplinary Approach*. New York: Elsevier; 1987.

Midanik L. The value of self reported alcohol consumption and alcohol problems: a literature review. *Br J Addict* 1982;77:357–82.

Sgroi S. *Handbook of Clinical Intervention in Child Sexual Abuse*. Lexington Mass: Lexington Books; 1982.

Slaughter L, Brown C, Crowley S, Peck R. Patterns of genital injury in female sexual assault victims. *Am J Obstet Gynecol* 1997;176:609–16.

Stark M, editor. *A Physician's Guide to Clinical Forensic Medicine*. Totowa, NJ; Humana Press; 2000.

Stockwell T, Stirling L. Estimating alcohol content of drinks: common errors in applying the unit system. *BMJ* 1989;298:571–2.

Sullivan JB, Hauptmann M, Bronstein AC. Lack of observable intoxication in humans with high plasma alcohol concentrations. *J Forensic Sci* 1987;32:1660–5.

The National Health Service Act 1977, The NHS Trusts and Primary Care Trusts (Sexually Transmitted Diseases) Directions 2000 revoking the 1991 directions.

Appendix 5.1
Pro forma for post-pubertal female and male forensic sexual assault examination

> **NOTE:** This form has been designed for use by Police Surgeons (also known as Forensic Medical Examiners, Forensic Physicians or Sexual Offence Examiners). It is provided to assist the examining doctor in the assessment of an adult complainant of sexual assault. It is to be regarded as an aide-memoire and it is therefore not necessary for all parts of the proforma to be completed. On completion this form is the personal property of the examining doctor.

1. EXAMINATION DETAILS

Location... Date of examination..

Time of arrival .... Time introduced to complainant.....................

2. DOCTOR DETAILS

Name of FME ....

Other doctors (if present) ....

GP details...

3. POLICE DETAILS

Name of attending police officer...

Name of investigating officer...

4. OTHERS PRESENT

Social worker/Care worker ....

Others (relationship to examinee) ....

5. PATIENT DETAILS

Name..

Date of Birth .... Age ....

Gender   FEMALE/MALE   Ethnicity ....

Marital status   Lives with ....

Occupation ....

6. CONSENT TO EXAMINATION AND REPORT

I .... consent to a medical examination as explained to

me by Dr .... to include:

a)   Full medical examination from top to toe
b)   Collection of forensic specimens/clothing
c)   Taking of photographs for record and evidential purposes
d)   Slides/videocolposcopic recording/diagnostic/training via a colposcope
e)   Consent for the use of anonymised data from this proforma to be used for
      medical research

I understand that Dr ....may have to
produce a report based on the examination and that details of the examination may
have to be revealed in court.

I have been advised that I may strike out any of the above before I sign and halt the
examination at any time.

I understand that the information recorded on this form and any photographs taken
may be later required by the court.

Signed... Date..

Signed... Date..

Name (& relationship of person with parental authority) ....

Witnessed...

Name of Witness ....

Relationship of witness ....

7. HISTORY of ASSAULT

Briefing taken from ....

Contact details ....

Location of assault...

History of events ....

....

....

....

....

....

Confirmation/additions from complainant (verbatim & recorded contemporaneously)

....

....

Are you aware of any injuries? (Details)

....

....

Are you aware of any ano-genital bleeding? ....

....

Weapon Used?   YES/NO: (Details)

....

Damage to clothing? YES/NO: (Details)

....

8.   OTHER SEXUAL ACTIVITIES

(details e.g. urinating, sucking or biting, spitting or ejaculating over body.)

....

....

Penis to mouth   yes/no   Penis to anus   yes/no

9.   DRUG AND ALCOHOL USE IN RELATION TO ASSAULT

	DATE	TIME	ALCOHOL	DRUG
5 days pre assault				
12hrs pre assault				
Post assault				

10. POST ASSAULT – ask if relevant

	YES	NO
Eaten	☐	☐
Drank	☐	☐
Wiped (specify site and disposal of e.g. cloth / tissue)	☐	☐
Bowels open	☐	☐
Passed urine (*note time*)	☐	☐
Changed clothes (*specify*)	☐	☐
Self harm (*sites*)	☐	☐
Complaints of pain/soreness/bleeding post assault	☐	☐

Details ....

Brushed teeth/gums/dentures (*circle*) Mouth wash/spray used (*circle*)

Washed/Bathed/Showered/Douched (*circle)*

Changed tampon/pad/sponge/diaphragm (*circle*)

Forensic samples taken before examination started:

Details ....

By whom taken ....

11. MEDICAL HISTORY

Past medical/surgical history/hospital admissions

....

....

....

....

....

....

....

....

....

Major psychiatric diagnoses...

Learning difficulties..

Suicidal/DSH..
Obstetric and gynaecological history

Present contraception... TAMPON/PAD USER ?

LMP.................................. Cycle.................... Menarche if relevant ....

Children .... Modes of delivery ....

Current genito-urinary symptoms

....

....

Past history vulvo-vaginal trauma / surgery

....

....

Current vulvo-vaginal skin disease / infection

....

Past history of anal trauma / surgery / bleeding on defaecation

....

Current anal skin disease / infection

....

Sexual history

SI prior to assault in last 14 days: YES/NO

If yes, note date:...

If yes, was condom used: ....

If yes, was lubricant used (*note type*):...

SI post assault: YES/NO

Types of intercourse in last 14 days only

....

....

Current drug history (this is defined as drugs used in last 5 days)
If recorded elsewhere e.g. "scenesafe form" no need to duplicate
Note strength and dosage and when medication was last taken

Prescribed...

....

....

....

OTC ....

....

....

Illicit ....

....

....

....

12. EXAMINATION

Name(s) of persons present ....

....

Height..

Weight...

Skin Colour..

Hair Colour..

Demeanour..

Disability (*note type*)

....

....

Head to Toe Survey
(detail below and on APS body diagrams when appropriate)

Notes inc. measurements, colour, shape, site, type of injury etc.
Document negative findings

Scalp/Hair

Face

Eyes

Ears

Lips

Inside mouth/Palate

Teeth

Neck

Back

Buttocks

Arms R /L

Hands/Wrists R/L

Fingers and Nails R/L (note if cut/broken/false/bitten)

Front of Chest

Breasts

Abdomen

Legs R / L

Feet/Ankles/Soles R/L

Additional details e.g. jewellery injuries, items lost at scene, injection sites/self harm

Other findings

SYSTEMS EXAMINATION
CVS

Pulse rate / character .... BP ....

Heart sounds ....

....

Other findings ....

RS

Trachea / Air entry / PN etc ....

Breath sounds... PEFR (if indicated) ....

Abdomen

L.K.K.S ....

Tenderness/Masses..

Bowel sounds...

Diagram (if indicated)

CNS

Pupil size and reactions..

Eye movement/nystagmus...

Conjunctivae ....

Conscious level...

Balance/Coordination..

Reflexes...

Genital Examination – tick as indicated

☐ Extra lighting   ☐ Colposcope   ☐ Additional magnification

☐ Position used – clarify: ....

Details of Female Genital Findings (and recorded on APS body diagrams)

Thighs

Pubic area

Pubic hair

Labia majora

Labia minora

Fourchette

Fossa Navicularis

Vestibule

Hymen (diagram when indicated)

Internal findings

Vaginal wall

Cervix

Size of speculum used: SMALL/MEDIUM/LARGE

Foley catheter used: YES/NO

Sterile water used: YES/NO   Lubricant used YES/NO Type:

Details of Male Genital Findings (and recorded on APS body diagrams)

Thighs

Pubic Area

Pubic Hair

Scrotum

Testes

Penis

Foreskin

Details of Anal Findings

Natal fold

Perianal/Anal margin

Internal findings

Proctoscope used : size and type :

Sterile water used: YES/NO   Lubricant used YES/NO   Type

Diagram (if indicated)

FORENSIC SAMPLES (If Scenesafe form or similar not used)

Identification number	Description of sample	Moistened Yes/No	Time taken

To whom handed ....

Date and Time samples handed over ....

After Care – include details

	YES	NO	DETAILS
Eaten	☐	☐	....
STD screening referral	☐	☐	....
PCC given / referral for IUCD	☐	☐	....
Antibiotics given	☐	☐	....
Other medication given	☐	☐	....
Referral for Hep B immunisation/PEP	☐	☐	....
Referral to GP	☐	☐	....
Referral to other support services	☐	☐	....
Post sexual assault leaflet given	☐	☐	....
Advice given to complainant	☐	☐	....

....

....

Time examination concluded...

Time notes concluded...

Dated and signed by FME ....

Witnessed notes made at time of examination...

Conclusions/Advice given to police:

Chapter 6

The general examination

Deborah Rogers

Aims and objectives

Patients who have been sexually assaulted may also have been physically assaulted or administered drugs or alcohol. In addition, they could have pre-existing physical illnesses, mental disorder or learning difficulties and they may have consumed drugs or alcohol voluntarily. In the context of an allegation of a sexual assault, the aim of the general examination is to document all the available medical and forensic evidence, in order to assist the court in its deliberations regarding the veracity of the allegation. This requires the forensic practitioner to remain objective and impartial even though the account of the assault may be particularly harrowing.

The objectives of the general examination can be summarised as:

- identification and retrieval of any stains, secretions, fibres, hairs or particles that could be relevant to a police investigation (see Chapter 7)
- identification and precise documentation of all injuries (fresh or healed) or abnormal signs that might relate to the alleged incident
- recognition and documentation of any pre-existing physical illnesses or evidence of mental disorder or learning difficulties
- identification and documentation of any signs of drug or alcohol use
- documentation of all negative findings; e.g. that all body surfaces were examined and no injuries or abnormalities noted.

Content

Although the forensic practitioner may feel under considerable pressure to obtain any relevant forensic samples, the general examination should commence with an initial appraisal of the patient's physical and emotional needs and of her mental state. If moderate to severe injuries are identified or other potentially serious medical or psychological conditions detected, it may be necessary to access the necessary secondary medical care before proceeding with the forensic assessment.

Following the initial appraisal, the general examination involves obtaining the relevant forensic samples (see Chapter 7) concurrent with the inspection, palpation, movement (in relation to the musculoskeletal system) and, if relevant, auscultation of the relevant body surfaces and systems. If drugs or alcohol may have been consumed in relation to the incident (and the patient presents within a timeframe whereby the effects of that substance may still be apparent) the pulse, blood pressure and central nervous system (including level of consciousness) must also be assessed. Where patients are known or believed to be suffering from a mental disorder, it is also necessary to conduct an assessment of the complainant's mental state.

Even when the allegation only relates to peno-oral penetration or genital touching, the patient should be offered a comprehensive examination of the non-intimate body surfaces. Failure to undertake a comprehensive general examination may result in asymptomatic injuries being overlooked that could corroborate the patient's account of the incident. Furthermore, a limited examination based on the complainant's account may be considered partisan, as it could potentially miss evidence that could corroborate the defendant's account of the encounter (e.g. a 'love bite').

Timing

It is standard procedure to offer a general examination to a patient who has been subjected to a 'recent' sexual assault. This is to ensure that any stains, secretions, fibres, hairs or particles that could be relevant to a police investigation are collected before they are removed and to enable precise documentation of all injuries that might relate to the alleged incident. It also enables the patient's urgent medical needs, in particular emergency contraception and sexually transmitted infection prophylaxis (see Chapter 9), to be addressed. There is no universally agreed definition of what constitutes a 'recent' sexual assault. The patient's medical needs, the nature of the allegation, the likelihood of detecting forensically important evidence (see Table 6.1) and the possibility of identifying injuries will determine the urgency of the examination. Ideally, the expediency of the examination should be determined on a case-by-case basis following consultation between an experienced forensic practitioner and the investigating officer.

Table 6.1 Persistence of spermatozoa

Site	Persistence of spermatozoa
Vagina	Up to seven days
Anal canal, rectum	Up to three days
Mouth	Up to two days
Skin	Not known; may persist after cleansing
Hair	Not known; may persist after cleansing

Place

In the UK, the majority of complainants of sexual assault are taken to designated examination suites. The police own most of these premises. Some are located in police stations (albeit separate from the custody areas) whereas others are in remote buildings. At best, these facilities are stocked with first-aid provisions. Therefore, they are not suitable for the management of patients with moderate to severe injuries. Such patients may need to be assessed and treated in a hospital accident and emergency department prior to the forensic examination.

In 1986, Dr Raine Roberts, a senior police surgeon in Manchester, developed the first sexual assault referral centre in the UK. The centre is known as the St Mary's Centre. It is located within the main building of the Women's and Children Hospital, Manchester, and, although staffed by forensic healthcare professionals, it affords the full support of the hospital staff should the patient's condition deteriorate or a moderate or severe injury be identified. Similar centres have been opened at Kings College Hospital, London (The Haven), on the site of the Royal Preston Hospital, Lancashire (The SAFE Centre), and REACH in Sunderland and Newcastle.

On occasion, a police officer may form the view that it is unnecessary to transport the patient from the police station to a specialist suite; this particularly arises in relation to complainants of indecent assault where the police officer perceives that only a limited examination is necessary. If asked to conduct a limited general examination of a complainant of sexual assault in the medical room of a police station (in the custody area), the forensic practitioner must decide how comprehensive the examination should be and determine that there is no possibility of cross-contamination (suspects are also examined in these rooms). Finally, the doctor must consider the distress that the patient may experience in the environs of a busy custody area and balance this with any inconvenience that a transfer may cause the patient. The patient's views on these matters will be pertinent to this decision.

Types of general injuries

Bruises, abrasions, incisions, lacerations and erythema have all been identified on complainants of sexual assault during the forensic medical examination.[1] The different terms reflect the macroscopic appearance of the injury and the method of causation.

Bruises

Bruises are caused by trauma to blood vessels that allows the blood normally contained therein to spread into the surrounding tissues. This blood and its subsequent breakdown may cause discoloration of the skin. Although bruises originate at the site of the trauma, those that develop in lax subcutaneous tissues may shift, under the influence of gravity, to appear elsewhere on the body. An example of this is when the patient sustains a single blow to the centre of the forehead and the blood gravitates to both periorbital areas, giving the false impression that more than one blow has been sustained. Similarly, bruises which originate in deep tissues may appear later at a distant site due to tracking along fascial planes and deflection by anatomical structures.

The extent of any bruising will depend upon the number of blood vessels that are disrupted (which in turn relates to vessel fragility, mass and velocity of impact), the laxity or otherwise of the surrounding tissues (fibrous subcutaneous tissue; e.g. on the palms, scalp and soles, limits the development of a bruise) and the efficiency of the patient's clotting mechanism. The variability of these factors means that it is not possible to determine conclusively the degree of force that has been applied to cause a given bruise.

As discussed above, some bruises may not be visible initially on the skin surface. In such cases, the presence of bruising may be suggested by tenderness on the overlying body surface. However, it is recognised that tenderness is a subjective finding which has a variety of causes. Forensic practitioners are advised to distract the patient while palpating the relevant body surfaces and where possible return to the 'tender' area later in the consultation to confirm its location. Even so, courts may consider evidence of tenderness to be 'hearsay' evidence and refuse to hear it. The Court may be more prepared to admit evidence of tenderness if bruising subsequently develops at the tender site.

There are anecdotal accounts that some individuals bruise easily. This is certainly the case in the elderly, who have increased blood-vessel fragility to the extent that even minor blows can result in extensive bruising. Knight expresses the view that fat people bruise more easily than thin ones "because of the greater volume of subcutaneous tissues" in the former. This view has not been verified by research and appears to contradict Knight's view that "children tend to bruise more easily than adults presumably because of the softer tissues and the smaller volume of protecting tissue that overlies the vessels".[2]

On occasions, patients will colour the skin in order to mimic or exaggerate bruising. This is usually apparent as the ink, dye or make-up tends to concentrate in the skin folds and pores. If this is suspected, the 'bruise' should be wiped with a moistened swab or tissue; if the colour is lifted the swab or tissue should be retained as forensic evidence.

Petechial haemorrhages

Petechial haemorrhages are small bruises typically defined as less than 2 mm in diameter.[3] In practice, it is extremely difficult macroscopically to measure precisely lesions that are less than 2 mm in size. On occasions, petechial haemorrhages merge to form a larger bruise.

Some commentators state that petechial haemorrhages are areas of 'peri-capillary bleeding',[3] whereas others state that "capillary bleeding would only be visible under a microscope and even petechiae originate from a larger order blood vessel than a capillary".[4]

Petechial haemorrhages can be identified on the skin, mucous membranes and serous membranes or on the cross-sectional surface of an organ. They are caused by:

- increased pressure in the blood vessels, e.g. strangulation, mechanical asphyxia, persistent coughing or vomiting; in strangulation and mechanical asphyxia, the petechiae develop above the site of the constriction
- dragging of the skin, e.g. oblique blunt trauma and suction of the skin; the latter is seen in relation to 'love bites'
- blunt trauma through woven fabrics
- medical diseases, e.g. vasculitis.

It is not known, and will probably never be known, how long pressure must be applied to the neck before petechial haemorrhages appear in the eyelids, conjunctiva and facial skin.[5] It is also not known whether concurrent factors that can increase venous pressure, such as struggling and screaming, expedite the development of petechial haemorrhages in such circumstances. However, it is widely accepted that pressure on the baroreceptors in the carotid sinuses, the carotid sheaths and the carotid body may cause a bradycardia (which presumably may produce loss of consciousness) and cardiac arrest without causing any petechial haemorrhages.

In the living, petechial haemorrhages disappear rapidly, although it is not possible to give a precise timescale for this.

Abrasions

Abrasion (colloquially referred to as a graze or scratch) is the term used to describe superficial disruptions of the surface epithelium (epidermis) caused by trauma. Some texts state that an abrasion is the result of damage to the epidermis alone and, thus, an abrasion does not bleed. This definition is controversial as even superficial injuries may bleed, because of the undulating architecture of the epidermal–dermal junction, in which the blood vessels are contained. Furthermore, adherence to this definition leaves a void with regard to the term that should be used to describe a deeper injury which otherwise has all the features of an abrasion. Some practitioners use the term 'laceration' in that situation.

Usually the causative force is applied tangentially to the skin but abrasions may also be due to perpendicular force. In the former, the epidermis may be lifted at the point of contact but remain intact distal to the point of contact, leaving a tag of skin. This is helpful in terms of determining the direction of the trauma. In other instances the epithelium may be transferred onto the causative object: this transfer can provide useful information in terms of linking an object or surface to the injury. In both circumstances fragments from an object or surface may remain in the wound, again providing forensic evidence.

Lacerations

Lacerations are splits in the skin. On the general body surfaces they are caused by blunt trauma. The typical features of a laceration caused by blunt trauma are irregular wound edges, bruised and abraded wound margins and tissue bridges (nerves and blood vessels) within the wound.

Incised wounds

Incised wounds are breaches in the epithelium caused by sharp objects. They are colloquially called 'cuts' as they are produced as the sharp object incises or cuts through the skin. Typically, incised wounds have straight edges, which are devoid of bruises or abrasions, and they have no tissue bridges (compare with lacerations). However, when the 'sharp' object is in fact blunt or irregularly shaped, the wound edges may be bruised and abraded and the wound may be irregular, making it difficult to determine the precise cause of the injury. In such cases the forensic practitioner should concentrate on describing the wound in detail rather than trying to categorise it.

Incised wounds may be further subdivided into slashes (length greater than depth) and stabs (depth greater than length). Although the history and appearance may suggest a stab wound, the wound must be explored to definitively reach this conclusion. As it is often difficult to determine the depth of a wound by observation alone, 'stab' wounds should be referred for exploration to exclude involvement of deeper tissues.

Erythema

Erythema (or reddening) of the skin may develop within seconds of the injury as a part of the 'triple response'. It may also appear later as part of the healing process (typically at the wound edges) or because of secondary infection. In these circumstances, the erythema is due to vasodilatation of the blood vessels and, as such, will blanch if compressed.

Erythema has multiple causes that include simple pressure on the skin (for example sitting on a chair) and skin diseases. In the former, the erythema will disappear when the pressure is removed. In the latter, the erythema may not blanch. This could cause an inexperienced practitioner to misinterpret the erythema as bruising.

Documentation of injuries

All injuries (fresh or healed) that might relate to the alleged incident must be documented in terms of their site in relation to a fixed anatomical point and adjacent injuries, size, colour (including whether it blanches) or the covering surface (e.g. blood, scab). If the skin has been breached the following should also be noted: depth of the wound, structures (if any) visible in the base of the wound, degree of blood loss, foreign material in the wound, orientation of skin tags and the wound edges. This information must be recorded in the contemporaneous notes, ideally on body diagrams. Complicated injury patterns, extensive injuries that challenge accurate recording and injuries that might have been caused by teeth or footwear must be photographed by a professional photographer.

Typically, the injuries are documented with the patient in the anatomical position. However, it may be more relevant, particularly in relation to the arms, to note the site of the injury when the patient assumes the position that they state they were in when they sustained the injury.

Many forensic practitioners choose to take photographs of the injuries they identify as an adjunct to their contemporaneous notes. These photographs may then be presented as part of the forensic evidence and, with the permission of the patient, used for teaching. Some police forces disapprove of this practice, so the forensic practitioner should obtain the permission of a police officer before obtaining any photographs. Photographs obtained by an amateur photographer do not obviate the need to obtain professional photographs when relevant. Courts accept digital photographs as evidence, although the photographer or any user should be prepared to demonstrate that the evidence is authentic and has not been manipulated. Well-documented procedures and written or electronic audit trails facilitate this. The images should be transferred to a WORM (Write Once Read Many) medium (e.g. a CD-R) as soon as possible after capture. A master copy, treated as any other evidence, must be stored safely. Working copies of the image files may be prepared, transferred, enhanced, etc., as required. Provided that the security is adequate, there is no reason why a master file could not be stored on an archive and retrieval system with electronic protection to alert to any manipulation to, and monitor access to, the file.[6]

Ageing injuries

It is impossible to age most injuries accurately. The best that can be stated is that the colour or state of healing of the injury is consistent with it having occurred at the time of the alleged incident.

The research by Langlois and Gresham demonstrated that, in photographs of bruises on people aged between ten and 100 years, the bruises may appear yellow as soon as 18 hours after the injury occurred.[7] Stephenson and Bialas noted similar findings in his study of the colour change of bruises in children aged eight months to 13 years.[8] However, the converse is not true: a bruise that is more than 18 hours old does not necessarily appear yellow. The Langlois and Gresham study also found that bruises on a single individual, caused at the same time in the same manner, could progress through different colour changes. This makes it difficult to relatively age multiple bruises on a given individual. No research has been undertaken regarding the ageing of bruises on dark skin.

The dilemmas

In the UK, the conviction rate for rape is very low.[9] A number of studies have found that, at the initial stage of an investigation, the presence of injuries is interpreted as 'evidence of violence' which correlates with a positive initial reaction from the legal authorities.[9-11] The significance given to injuries during the trial is more varied. Whereas one study found that evidence of trauma was significantly associated with a successful prosecution,[12] others found little correlation between the severity of the injuries and the judicial outcome.[13,14] Nonetheless, as previously stated, the aim of the general examination is to document all the available medical and forensic evidence in order to assist the court in its deliberations. Therefore, the first part of this section will consider whether it is possible to enhance the quality and quantity of the medical (and forensic) evidence by conducting a second examination or using alternative light sources.

Having identified and documented all the injuries, forensic practitioners may be asked to interpret them or comment on whether a lack of injuries negates the allegation. These dilemmas will be considered in the second half of this section.

Can second examinations enhance the quality and quantity of the medical evidence?

While an early examination is clearly pertinent in terms of collecting forensic evidence and documenting minor injuries that may rapidly disappear, some bruises may not develop for days.[15] However, second examinations are not part of routine forensic practice. It is not known how frequently second examinations would reveal injuries that were not present at the initial consultation, nor is it known how acceptable second examinations would be to the complainant. Furthermore, it is controversial whether a court would admit evidence of injuries gathered during a second examination, as it could be considered that the complainant may have self-inflicted bruises in the intervening time. Notwithstanding the potential controversies, most forensic practitioners advise complainants to inform the investigating officer if they develop any bruises in the first few days following the assault, so that the injury can be properly recorded.

Are alternative light sources a useful adjunct to the general examination?

The visible light spectrum ranges from violet light (420 nm) to red light (750 nm). Rays beyond the violet end of the spectrum are called ultraviolet rays (10 to about 420 nm) and rays beyond the red end of the spectrum are infrared rays (750 nm to about 1 mm). A Wood's lamp incorporates a filter so that it emits a high intensity, 'completely harmless' ultraviolet light of approximately 320–420 nm.[16] Use of electronic equipment, photography and special filters may extend the sensitivity of the human eye into the ultraviolet and infrared ends of the spectrum.

Many substances will adsorb light at one wavelength and emit it at another; this phenomenon is known as fluorescence. Although some types of fluorescence are visible to the human eye, in most cases narrow-band light sources and special filtered goggles are required to observe the effect.

It has been suggested that alternative light sources may have some uses in relation to the general (and genital) examination of a complainant of a sexual assault. These are considered below.

Identification of semen

One textbook advocates the use of Wood's lamp or 'an alternative light source' to scan the entire body in a darkened room in order to identify (and swab) stains that may be saliva, semen, vaginal fluid and blood.[1] However, a study by Santucci et al.[17] found that, while many creams and ointments fluoresced when exposed to a Wood's lamp (wavelength 360 nm), none of 28 semen samples did. Other authors have commented on the fact that detergents, lubricants (particularly those that contain petroleum jelly) and milk also fluoresce.[18]

However, when semen stains are exposed to a high-intensity light source of variable wavelengths (e.g. the Polilight®, manufactured by Rofin Australia Pty Ltd, Dingley Victoria, Australia) and viewed using goggles to cut out the strong excitation light, then semen may be detectable, even when the background surface is fluorescent.[19] Furthermore, the location of the stain may be recorded using photography.

An experiment by Marshall et al.[20] found that semen from a single donor could be detected on live skin using a large number of excitation wavelengths (emitted by a Poliray®, Rofin Australia Pty Ltd) and emission filter combinations. Optimal results were obtained using 415 nm ± 40 nm band-pass filter and a 475 high-pass and 505 band-pass ± 40 nm interference filter. Further research is to be undertaken using semen from multiple donors and in isolating semen from other fluorescing contaminates, e.g. oils.

Ultraviolet photography of injuries

Ultraviolet rays penetrate the superficial layers of the skin where, essentially, they are either absorbed or reflected. Following an injury, the healing process affects the way that ultraviolet light is absorbed and reflected. These changes may be recorded photographically using special equipment, even some time after the visible signs of the injury have disappeared. This technique is only suitable for demarcated injuries, such as bite marks, ligature marks, shoe marks and burns that can be related to an object.

Ultraviolet photography is not a replacement for standard photography of a fresh injury. However, on occasions the significance of a fresh injury may initially not be appreciated or other factors, such as bruising and swelling, may distort the fresh injury to a degree that it is not possible to make meaningful comparisons with an object or dental impression. Furthermore, some complainants may not present for several weeks after the alleged assault.

The optimum timing for photography is not known, although there is some evidence that ultraviolet photographs obtained in the first 12 hours may be of higher clarity than either colour or black and white photographs.[16] There is then a latent period (approximately 17 days) when no injury shows using ultraviolet photography, although bruising may be apparent to the naked eye.[16] The injury then reappears on ultraviolet photography and persists for two to five months, even though it is scarcely apparent to the naked eye.[16,21] It is suggested that reappearance and disappearance of the injury depends upon the severity of the injury and the rate of healing.[21]

This technique cannot be used to screen for injuries as, under ultraviolet light, nonspecific pigmentation of the skin can sometimes appear as dark.[22] Furthermore, the technique works much better on white skin than on black. It must be remembered that the absence of a demonstrable injury, even using ultraviolet photography, does not mean that a physical assault did not take place.

Identification of fresh injuries

Lynnerup and Hjalgrim[23] advocate the routine use of ultraviolet light in medico-legal examinations to evaluate stains and skin trauma. They describe the fluorescence of 'lesions of the skin' using a hand-held ultraviolet light with a wavelength of 321 nm in a dark room. It is stated that these 'lesions' represented bruising and swelling. However, before embarking on the routine screening advocated by these authors, a more comprehensive study that would take account of the fluorescence of non-traumatic skin lesions and skin disorders needs to be undertaken.

West et al.[24] used a high intensity, tuneable alternative light source to identify or enhance injuries on both the living and the dead. They used four narrow-band wavelengths (450 nm, 485 nm, 525 nm and 570 nm, each about

30 nm wide) and two wideband wavelengths (white light and all wavelengths less than 530 nm). The detected injuries were not only visible to the examiner (enhanced using coloured lenses in goggles) but could also be recorded on film using a 35 mm camera. West *et al.* had best success using the 450 wavelength and yellow lenses as band-pass filters.

Changes in the thermal conductivity of the skin occur in response to disease processes. Infrared thermography has applications in rheumatology, orthopaedics and oncology. It has also been used to detect and monitor burns and skin ulcers. It is not known whether this technology could be applied to clinical forensic medicine to detect fresh injuries that are not discernible externally.

Clearly, alternative light sources may have a role in the general (and genital) examination of a complainant of sexual assault. However, before advocating the routine use of alternative light sources, more information is needed regarding the optimum excitation wavelengths and emission filters to detect semen, other body fluids and injuries, the specificity of the recommended method and any health and safety implications for both the examiner and examinee, as short wavelength (200–300 nm) ultraviolet light can damage the eye.[16] Finally, before such evidence could be relied on in court, there would need to be a comprehensive study to determine whether old injuries were also highlighted by alternative light sources.

Interpretation of the injuries

More than 50% of all complainants of sexual assaults have general injuries noted at the time of the examination, most of which are minor (e.g. bruises, abrasions and erythema for which no specific intervention is required).[25–27] However, minor general injuries may be sustained as part of normal daily activities. Therefore, because of the difficulty in ageing injuries precisely it may not be possible to relate injuries definitively to an alleged sexual assault.

There are anecdotal reports that consensual sexual intercourse may result in minor general injuries such as bites, scratches and bruises.[28] Currently, there are no available data to distinguish minor general injuries sustained during consensual sexual activity from those sustained following nonconsensual sexual activity. Therefore, even when the colour or state of healing of a minor injury makes it consistent with having been caused at the time of the alleged incident it does not mean that the sexual act was nonconsensual.

Moderate (e.g. lacerations that requiring suturing, large bruises and facial and extremity fractures that do not require hospitalisation) and severe injuries clearly may have more significance and need to be adequately explained.[29] Patterned injuries (which demonstrate the shape or indentations in an object) or injuries at certain sites may also be more significant; for example, patterned abrasions and bruises around the wrists caused by physical restraints.

When considering any injury or collection of injuries one must consider whether there is any indication that they may have been self-inflicted. Typically, self-inflicted injuries are superficial incised wounds that run parallel to one another, do not cross sensitive areas (such as eyes, lips and ears) and are within reach of the dominant hand.[30] However, there are case reports of abrasions and excoriations having been self-inflicted.[31]

Does the absence of medical findings negate an allegation?

Although there are many papers that describe the general injuries to complainants of sexual assault, there are only a limited number that relate the type of sexual assault to the frequency and severity of general injuries. Some papers have identified factors that are associated with an increased likelihood of sustaining general injuries during a sexual assault.[32-35] These include:

- older complainants
- there was also a physical assault
- there was anal penetration
- the complainant physically resisted
- the offender had a weapon
- there was more than one offender.

However, this does not mean that complainants who describe these circumstances will necessarily sustain injuries, as there are so many compounding variables such as the amount of force used. Nonetheless, barristers frequently invite forensic practitioners to state that he/she would have expected to see an injury or injuries if the sexual assault had occurred in the manner alleged by the complainant. However, such statements only reflect the practitioner's opinion and, because it is not possible to reproduce the circumstances of each alleged sexual assault, do not have any scientific foundation.

Conclusion

It is essential that complainants of sexual assault are offered a comprehensive general examination, during which all injuries, potentially significant scars and medical conditions are noted and the necessary forensic samples are obtained. Alternative light sources may be a useful adjunct to the general examination in terms of detecting body fluids and identifying (and recording) fresh and old injuries. However, more research needs to be done in this field before they are recommended for routine use. There also needs to be more research comparing the general injuries noted among complainants of sexual assault with those noted among the general population.

References

1. Girardin BW, Faugno DK, Seneski PC, Slaughter L, Whelan M. *Color Atlas of Sexual Assault.* St Louis MI: Mosby;1997.
2. Knight B. *Forensic Pathology.* 2nd ed. London: Arnold; 1996. p. 141–2.
3. Jaffe F. Petechial hemorrhages – A review of pathogenesis. *Am J Forensic Med Pathol* 1994;15:203–7.
4. Knight B. *Forensic Pathology*, 2nd ed. London: Arnold; 1996. p. 140.
5. Knight B. *Forensic Pathology*, 2nd ed. London: Arnold; 1996. p. 364.
6. Sheila Hardwick, Police Scientific Development Branch. Personal Communication.
7. Langlois N, Gresham G. The ageing of bruises: a review and study of the colour changes with time. *Forensic Sci Int* 1991;50:227–38.
8. Stephenson T, Bialas Y. Estimation of the age of bruising. *Arch Dis Child* 1996;74:53–5.
9. Harris J, Grace S. *A Question of Evidence Investigating and Prosecuting Rape in the 1990s.* Home Office Research Study no. 196. London: Home Office; 1999.
10. Helweg-Larson K. The value of the medico-legal examination in sexual offences. *Forensic Sci Int* 1985;27:145–55.
11. Penttila A, Karhumen PJ. Medicolegal findings among rape victims. *Med Law* 1999;9:329–37.
12. Rambow B, Adkinson C, Frost T, Peterson G. Female sexual assault: medical and legal implications. *Ann Emerg Med* 1992;21:727–31.
13. Helweg-Larson K. The value of the medico-legal examination in sexual offences. *Forensic Sci Int* 1985;27:145–55.
14. Penttila A, Karhumen PJ. Medicolegal findings among rape victims. *Med Law* 1999;9:329–37.
15. Knight B. *Forensic Pathology.* 2nd ed. London: Arnold; 1996. p. 142.
16. West M, Billings J, Frair J. Ultra-violet photography: bite marks on human skin and suggested technique for the exposure and development of reflective ultra-violet photography. *J Forensic Sci* 1987;32:1204–13.
17. Santucci K, Nelson D, Kemedy K, McQuillen K, Duffy S, Linakis J. Wood's lamp utility in the identification of semen. *Pediatrics* 1999;104:1342–4.
18. Jones D. The task of the Forensic Science Laboratory in the investigation of sexual offences. *J Forensic Sci Soc* 1963;3:88–93.
19. Stoilovic M. Detection of semen and blood stains using Polilight as a light source. *Forensic Sci Int* 1991;51:289–296.
20. Marshall S, Bennett A, Fravel H. Locating semen on live skin using visible fluorescence. Paper presented at the Sixth International Conference in Clinical Forensic Medicine of the World Police Medical Officers, Sydney, Australia, March 17–22, 2002.
21. Krauss T, Warlen S. The forensic science use of reflective ultra-violet photography. *J Forensic Sci* 1985;30:262–8.
22. Creer K. Personal communication.
23. Lynnerup N, Hjalgrim H. Routine use of ultraviolet light in medico-legal examinations to evaluate stains and skin trauma. *Med Sci Law* 1995;35:165–8.
24. West M, Barsley R, Hall J, Hayne S, Cimrmancic M. The detection and documentation of trace wound patterns by use of an alternative light source. *J Forensic Sci* 1992;37:1480–8.
25. Riggs N, Houry D, Long G, Markovchick V, Feldhaus K. Analysis of 1076 cases of sexual assault. *Ann Emerg Med* 2000;35:358–62.
26. Bowyer L, Dalton M. Female victims of rape and their genital injuries. *Br J Obstet Gynaecol* 1997;104:617–20.
27. Bottomly C, Sadler T, Welch J. Integrated clinical service for sexual assault victims in a genito-urinary setting. *Sex Transm Infect* 1999;75:116–19.
28. Helweg-Larson K. The value of the medico-legal examination in sexual offences. *Forensic Sci Int* 1985;27:145–55.
29. Tintinalli J, Hoelzer M. Clinical findings and legal resolution in sexual assault. *Ann Emerg Med* 1951;4:447–51.
30. Knight B. *Forensic Pathology.* 2nd ed. London: Arnold; 1996. p. 238.
31. Faller-Marquardt M, Ropohl D, Pollak S. Excoriations and contusions of the skin as artefacts in fictitious sexual offences. *J Clin Forensic Med*1995;2:129–36.

32.   Ruback R, Ivie D. Prior relationship, resistance and injury in rapes: an analysis of crisis centre records. *Violence Vict* 1988;3:99–111.
33.   Mori C. Patterns of violence in sexual assault of adults. Medical student elective project. Unpublished data.
34.   Slaughter L, Brown CRV, Crowley S, Peck R. Patterns of genital injury in female sexual assault victims. *Am J Obstet Gynecol* 1997;176:609–16.
35.   Wright R, West D. Rape – a comparison of group offences and lone assaults. *Med Sci Law* 1981;21:25–30.

Chapter 7

The sexual assault medical examination kit

Mary Newton

Introduction

Few other criminal offences require as extensive an examination and collection of evidence as that of a sexual assault. There are many types of sexual assault, only some of which involve penetration of a body cavity. The provision of a sexual assault kit is paramount in the investigation process as it serves to provide the practitioner with the relevant samples to retrieve and preserve forensic evidence. The samples collected may eliminate a suspect, identify an assailant and substantiate an allegation, which in turn may lead to a prosecution. It is therefore important not only that the evidence is collected properly but that the kit itself provides for the appropriate collection of evidence.

The kit should contain sufficient samples to allow the practitioner to undertake a top-to-toe examination where the allegation warrants it and clear guidance on what samples should be taken and why. The guidelines should act as a reference to enable the practitioner to focus on specific sample collection and thus respect the examinee. Reactions to sexual assault vary widely and the forensic examination may be difficult for the patient. Parts of the examination may have to be omitted or deferred unless medically indicated. Only doctors and nurses who have acquired specialist knowledge and training should use the sexual assault kit. If a law enforcement agency requests a forensic medical examination of a complainant or a suspect of an alleged sexual assault it is usual for the agency to pay the cost of the medical examination kit.

The first part of this chapter endeavours to guide the practitioner through use of the kit. Information provided includes reasons for sampling, methods of collection and preservation of forensic evidence from an adult complainant or a suspect of a sexual assault, so that the medical examination is as through, timely and respectful as current knowledge and capacity allow. Reference to the persistence data mentioned in the purpose and reasons for each of the modules will help the forensic practitioner to determine whether the forensic examination of a complainant should be conducted out of office hours or could be deferred until the next day. For example, in a stranger assault where the complainant describes being restrained by the offender, the timing of the examination should be influenced by the speed with which clinical signs such as reddening on the skin will fade (see Swab module, skin swabbing).

A National Medical Examination Kit Working Party was formed in 1998 to bring together medical, law enforcement and forensic science committees in the form of the Association of Police Surgeons, the Association of Chief Police Officers and the Forensic Science Service. The Working Party members represent extensive experience and expertise working with cases of adult and child sexual assault. The modular kit outlined is endorsed by them and is currently used by 25 police forces in the UK.

The practical aspects of which samples to obtain and how to obtain them, and the clinical details required by the forensic scientist are addressed in each module section.

Basic scientific principles for the collection and analysis of forensic samples

The containers, instruments and swabs used to collect forensic evidence differ from those used in clinical tests. Only sealed, disposable instruments (e.g. scissors, forceps, nail clippers should be used when retrieving forensic samples.[1] If specula, proctoscopes or swabs require lubrication then only the sterile water samples provided should be used for this purpose (see Swab module below) The quality and integrity of all components in the kit must be ensured and must meet a minimum scientific standard.

Packaging and continuity

The integrity of the sexual assault kit specimens collected must be accounted for from the moment of collection until the time it is introduced in to a court of law as evidence. This process is necessary in order to maintain the legally necessary chain of evidence'.

Any retrieved items using the kit must be labelled and then packaged quickly and efficiently to prevent accidental loss of material and to minimise decomposition of the sample. Labelling the sample with a number reflecting the order in which the samples were obtained is particularly important when more than one sample has been obtained from the same site.[2] The kit contains clear bags with integral tamper-evident seals as proof that the sample has not been contaminated with exogenous substances since it was sealed. The bags also have integral labels so information referring to the contained exhibit does not become detached during sample storage.

Storage of samples

It is recommended that all samples in the medical examination kit are stored frozen until transport to the forensic laboratory for analysis. The exception to freezing applies to the alcohol, drugs, blood and urine collection modules.[3] These should be refrigerated if analysis is likely to be undertaken within six weeks of sampling. Correct storage is required to inhibit deterioration and to assure the best possible test results from the samples.

Kit storage box

The container should be robust, restockable and contain all the listed modules on the kit contents list. An outer identification label and integrity seals should be present.[4,5] There should be a visible expiry date on the box that relates to the modular contents. The manufacturers of the module components govern the expiry date. The kit should not be used if the date is beyond the expiry date or the integrity seals are not intact.

The Association of Police Surgeons has produced a leaflet about the services that are currently available to a complainant after the medical has been completed.[6] This leaflet is included in the documentation module. The leaflet includes information on sexual health, emergency contraception and options available with regard to advice and support. The forensic practitioner's name and the date of the medical examination should be completed and the leaflet given to the complainant.

The Association of Chief Police Officers Council has produced a booklet explaining the duty of care that the police have to a complainant who reports a sexual assault to them.[7] The booklet also provides a brief outline explaining the medical examination, what happens if there is a court case and how the complainant might feel as a result of the assault. Contact details for the police officers dealing with the case should be recorded in the booklet and provided for the complainant to read as soon as the allegation is reported.

Kit information and sampling guidelines (labelled as Medical Information 1 & 2) are provided, which give a checklist for the practitioner to follow when using the medical examination kit. Familiarity with the guidelines and contents of the kit on the part of the practitioner will facilitate examination of the patient.

The forensic scientist must be provided with salient information regarding the incident and what, if any, subsequent activities the complainant and suspect performed prior to the medical examination. Such activities include bathing, urination, defecation and brushing of teeth, any of which could help to explain the absence of body fluids or other foreign materials. Information provided will be used to assess the case and to aid in determining the order, type of forensic analysis and the number of samples to be examined. This in turn will help with the interpretation of any findings.

Evidence from the offender and the crime scene often may be found on the body and clothing of the complainant. When a prompt forensic medical examination takes place the chances increase that some type of physical evidence may be found. Conversely, the chances of finding physical evidence decrease in proportion to the length of time which elapses between the assault and the medical examination.

The MEDX tricarbonated pro formas are provided to record the information in a standardised format and should help the practitioner to focus on collection of those details relevant to the alleged offence and on the samples to be taken. Attempts to obtain too detailed a history of the incident at this stage, particularly when the patient may be feeling particularly vulnerable, may conflict with those details collected in subsequent statements, which may jeopardise the case at trial.[8] It should also be noted that the complainant would normally have provided details relating to the allegation to another professional, such as a police officer or crisis worker, prior to the forensic medical examination taking place. These details can be provided to the forensic practitioner by the third party and then clarified, if necessary, with the patient.

Form MEDX 1A is used to record information provided by the complainant specific to the alleged offence. When analysing body fluid specimens in sexual assault cases, the forensic laboratory sometimes identifies genetic markers that are inconsistent with a mixture of DNA from only the patient and the offender. For this reason, one of the questions asked of the complainant relates to the date and time of other relevant sexual activity within the previous ten days. The police may have to obtain elimination DNA sample from the partner if the laboratory subsequently advises that this is necessary (see DNA 2 buccal scrape module). If a condom was used during the sexual assault it is also important that a record is made of any use of a condom with regard to recent previous intercourse, i.e. within 30 hours for a female complainant.

Form MEDX 1B is used to record information that relates to samples that are collected from a complainant or suspect during a forensic medical examination (one per person). The pro forma records the number of samples taken, the module used and the exhibit identification mark (usually formed by the practitioner's initials and a number reflecting the order in which the samples listed were obtained). This form also records whether a speculum and or proctoscope were used during the examination. A continuation sheet (MEDX 1C) is provided should further information need to be recorded that is not captured on MEDX 1B.

Couch cover module

A free-size, protective cover for the medical examination couch is primarily provided to be used as a barrier between the complainant and the couch itself if an anogenital examination is required. The cover also aids the collection of particulate and physical evidence that may be present on the complainant's body. The cover should be placed over the couch before the examination takes place. On completion of the medical examination the cover should be folded inwards and placed in a labelled, tamper-evident bag and stored dry until transported to the forensic laboratory.

Disposable clothing module

This is to provide a groundsheet for the complainant to undress on, together with a free-size paper gown and pair of pants to be worn by the complainant once the clothing has been removed. The clothing that the complainant presents in is normally collected as she undresses while standing on the ground sheet. Once removed, the clothing is packaged individually by a person trained in the knowledge of forensic packaging; this should be someone other than the forensic practitioner. The clothing worn by the complainant during the assault or even subsequent to the incident may be an invaluable source of information in terms of the nature of the sexual assault, e.g. damage and distribution of body fluid stains, and the identification of the assailant.

The groundsheet primarily acts as a barrier between the complainant and the floor but also allows collection of particulate evidence from the scene and physical evidence, such as hairs from the assailant. The gown and pants are provided as modesty garments. In practice, the gown is used but the pants are only worn if the complainant has no change of clothing with her.

The groundsheet should be placed on the floor beyond the screen, within the area in which the complainant undresses. The complainant should be instructed to disrobe while standing on the groundsheet. To avoid contamination, only the complainant should handle her own clothing, if possible.

Once the complainant has undressed and handed individual items of clothing to the person nominated to package them, the groundsheet should be folded inward and placed in a labelled, tamper-evident bag and stored dry until transported to the forensic laboratory. After the complainant has redressed, the gown and paper pants, if worn, should be individually packaged in labelled, tamper-evident bags and stored dry until transported to the forensic laboratory.

Body outline module

For discussion of this module, see Chapter 8.

Mouth collection module

This is to collect samples within two days from the complainant where oral–penile contact has been made during a sexual assault or in circumstances in which details of the incident are unknown. Rapid retrieval of the forensic samples from the oral cavity is of paramount importance, due to the limited period that spermatozoa remain in this orifice. Only a few sperm are detected unless the sample is taken within a few hours of ejaculation.[9]

Patient distress is often apparent where fellatio is alleged. Although rinsing of the mouth, drinking and brushing of teeth do not necessarily remove all traces of spermatozoa,[10] such activities should be discouraged until this module has been used. For this reason, this module should be used as soon as possible after an allegation of nonconsensual fellatio is made.

To date, there are not sufficient results of studies investigating the order in which the samples should be taken. King *et al.*[11] reported a greater recovery of sperm from mouth rinsings against mouth swabs, recovering spermatozoa up to 13 hours after fellatio. It is therefore recommended that a mouth rinse should be routinely collected in these cases.[11] Samples can be collected by the patient herself, under the direction of a police officer or other attending professional, prior to the arrival of the forensic practitioner and minimising any delay.

Current practice in the UK is to obtain 10 ml saliva as the first sample in the container provided. Then two swabs in sequence are rubbed around the inside of the mouth, under the tongue and over the gum margins. Attention should be paid to those areas of the mouth, such as between the upper and lower lip, gum and along the gingiva, where spermatozoa might remain for the longest amount of time. If dentures or other dental fixtures are present these should be swabbed separately. The mouth is finally rinsed with the ampoule of 10 ml sterile water, which is provided. This should be collected in the container. The used ampoule should be retained together with the mouth rinse container. The saliva, sequential mouth swabs, mouth rinse container and the used ampoule are then placed in three separate labelled, tamper-evident bags. All three collected samples should be stored frozen until transported to the forensic laboratory. At the laboratory, the samples may be examined to identify spermatozoa followed by DNA analysis.

Hair sample collection module

This module is for sampling pubic and or head hair for possible contaminants. In a sexual assault, hair is most commonly sampled to detect body fluids. Although spermatozoa have been recovered from hair that was washed,[12] there are no detailed data regarding the persistence of spermatozoa on the hair in terms of time since assault.

Chemical analysis of recovered hairs may be relevant if the contamination is believed to be an exogenous substance such as a lubricant.[13] Precautionary combing of the pubic hair should routinely be carried out to retrieve foreign hairs or particles that may be transferred from one individual to the person or clothing of the other or the crime scene.[14] These hairs can be microscopically compared with known hair samples from both individuals to determine the origin. Discrimination of hair by microscopic means alone yields limited information in terms of assailant identification. Fluorescence *in situ* hybridisation (FISH) technology has been applied in a forensic setting to identify the gender of hair.[15] The research demonstrated that there was a potential application when considering the possible transfer of hair in sexual assault cases where microscopy cannot aid in determining the source.

Once the gender of the hair has been established, with the improved sensitivity provided by polymerase chain reaction (PCR) DNA techniques and the development of mitochondrial DNA analysis, stronger, more objective conclusions in terms of assailant identification can be reached.[16–18] Microscopic comparisons may also be employed in an attempt to identify any foreign particles recovered.

In the rare event that a balaclava or other article has been worn on the head during the assault, the presence of fibres in the head hair can provide strong evidence of contact with the article. Fibres have been recovered from the head hair even after washing up to seven days later.

Where there is evidence of semen or other matted material on pubic or head hair, it may be collected by cutting with the scissors provided. The cuttings and scissors should both be placed in a labelled, tamper-evident bag. It is important to obtain the complainant's permission prior to cutting any significant amount of contaminated hair. If the sample cannot be cut, it may be collected in the same manner as other dried fluid (see Swab module below) On occasion, both methods may be applicable. At the laboratory, analysis may be carried out to establish whether a body fluid is present, followed by DNA profiling.

Any foreign particles or hairs visibly identified on the head or pubic hair should be collected with the forceps provided and the material and the forceps placed on the drape provided which is folded inward. Good practice dictates that the absence of visible hairs or particles should also be noted on the MEDX 1B form. If the patient has no pubic or head hairs of their own visible, perhaps due to shaving, this should also be noted.

The complainant's pubic hairs should be routinely combed on to the second white drape provided, with the complainant lying on her side. Pubic hair combings may retrieve particulate evidence as well as extraneous hairs. It is therefore important that the comb in the kit is dark in colour and opaque, in order to facilitate the searching procedure at the forensic laboratory.[19] Complainants may prefer to do the combing themselves to reduce embarrassment and to increase their sense of control. The drape enclosing the comb should be folded inward and placed in a tamper-evident bag.

In addition to combing, a reference control sample should be taken from the suspect during the medical examination. The suggested method to reduce the discomfort for the suspect is cutting. A cut sample of 10–25 pubic hairs should be taken, as close to the skin as possible, and this fact recorded on form MEDX 1B (see Medical examination documentation module below), preferably with a note about the length of the remaining stubble.

In allegations where fibre contact may have occurred as a result of something being placed over the head, the head hair should be taped,[20] using the low-adhesive tape provided and the taping(s) attached to the acetate sheet provided. The acetate sheet should then be placed in the grip seal bag.

Any sample collected using the hair sample collection module should be placed in a separate, labelled, tamper-evident bag and stored frozen until transported to the forensic laboratory.

Fingernail sample collection module

These samples are used to collect potentially useful evidence of cross-transfer. During the course of a sexual assault, the patient will be in contact with the assailant as well as the environment. Trace materials such as skin,[21] body fluids, hairs, fibres and soil can collect under the fingernails of the patient. The incidence of cases submitted to the Forensic Science Service where digital penetration of the complainant by the offender had occurred was 18% in 2003. This act is often a precursor to penetration by a penis.

In 2003, the incidence of cases received by the Forensic Science Service where the complainant had scratched or pushed the offender away was 20%.[22] A number of DNA short tandem repeat (STR) results have been obtained from material recovered from fingernail samples of sexual assault complainants submitted to the Forensic Science Service. The results obtained demonstrate that it is possible to recover a secondary source of DNA even though the majority of material recovered originates from the donor's fingernails[23,24] These results mirror the work reported by several authors.[25,26] Lederer *et al.*[27] reported recovery of DNA matching the complainant's from a suspect's fingernails two days after the alleged digital penetration had occurred. The suspect denied any form of contact with the victim and also claimed to have washed his hands several times during this period of elapsed time.

It has also been observed that DNA profiles from unknown males have been obtained from several female murder victims even though their bodies had been submersed in water for different lengths of time.[28] In one case dealt with by the Forensic Science Service, a significant male profile was obtained from the fingernails of a dead prostitute six weeks after she went missing.[29] This demonstrates that fingernail samples should be considered, even if the complainant claims to have washed their hands after contact with the offender.

The complainant should be asked whether they had sustained contact with the offender's face, body or clothing. The contact may only be a scratch. If so, or if fibres or other materials are observed when the hands are examined, samples should be collected. Samples should also be considered if a fingernail broke during the assault, as the broken section may be retrievable. If the broken fragment is recovered, the residual nail should be clipped within 24 hours to enable both a mechanical fit and nail striation comparison to be performed at the laboratory.[30] If more than one nail is broken and it is not clear from which finger the broken nail came, clip and submit all the broken nails. Fingernail striations are individual to a particular finger.

Samples should be obtained from the suspect if it is alleged that his hands had direct contact with the genitalia. If there is any delay in the examination of the suspect, the hands should be protected in tamper-evident bags to prevent loss of evidence from washing or wiping etc.[31]

The method of sampling fingernails currently recommended is to take clippings of the whole fingernail, all nails on both hands. The clippers provided have a protective, sealed cover to contain the clippings. One of the white drapes from the module should be unfolded and placed on a flat surface. One hand should be held over the drape and the fingernails of sufficient length should be clipped using one of the pair of fingernail clippers. The process should then be repeated with the other hand. Clippings are more practical to handle for the forensic laboratory but, in some cases, the fingernails may be too short to cut or the complainant may withhold consent for the sample. In such cases, the nails should be scrapped with the plastic quills provided. It is important that scrapings are made for each hand over one of the white drapes. The drape should then be folded inward to contain the quill. Repeat the process with the other hand. Clipping or scraping is a procedure that the complainant may want to perform herself and she should be encouraged to do so.

Swab module

The swab module is for collecting samples from the female genitalia or from the skin where body fluids or lubricant may have been deposited. Swabs should be collected where the detection of semen from the female genitalia is required, up to seven days after sexual intercourse is alleged, and up to two days from the male genitalia where the detection of body fluids such as vaginal epithelial cells, saliva and blood are required. If anal intercourse has occurred, swabs should be collected up to three days after the act has occurred.

There are no published data as to how long body fluids persist on unwashed skin of the living and in particular for how long after deposit a DNA profile can be obtained. One Forensic Science Service biologist has obtained a DNA short tandem repeat (STR) profile matching the assailant from a swab of unwashed face skin of a sexual assault complainant who alleged the assailant slobbered over her face. The face swab was collected within six hours of the offence.[32]

The swabs provided in the module do not contain transport media, as they will only be analysed at a forensic laboratory. The swab tips are standard and have been selected to maximise both absorption and extraction characteristics for recovery purposes at the medical examination and then subsequently during laboratory examination.[33-35]

An ampoule of 10 ml sterile water is provided to moisten swabs used to sample dried material and to lubricate the speculum or proctoscope as required. At the end of the forensic assessment, the opened ampoule of sterile water should be placed in the container provided. The ampoule has recorded batch information and this can act as a quality control check for the water, if required, at the laboratory.

The Forensic Science Service is most often asked to check whether or not semen is present on intimate swabs collected from the female genitalia when penile-vaginal penetration is alleged in sexual assault cases. Microscopy is employed to identify spermatozoa and microscopy and electrophoretic techniques to identify seminal fluid where no spermatozoa are present.[36,37] Interpretation is also requested in the context of the case with regard to the quantity (determined crudely) and quality of spermatozoa present on intimate swabs in relation to time since intercourse.

It is important that the forensic practitioner samples the vagina, vulva and perineum separately when only anal intercourse is alleged by the female complainant, to exclude the possibility of leakage from the vagina accounting for semen in the anal canal, a question that the forensic laboratory can only address if the samples are collected and subsequently submitted for analysis.

Non-genital skin swabs may be required where ejaculation has occurred on the area or where epithelial cells may be deposited where kissing, biting, sucking or licking is alleged or where excessive contact has occurred, e.g. where attempted strangulation has occurred. While epithelial cells can be recognised by a competent microscopist, it should be emphasised that it is not possible, by microscopy alone, to establish from which orifice such cells may have originated. Such cellular material is amenable to DNA profiling techniques.[38]

In cases of cunnilingus or anilingus, a check will be made for the assailant's DNA on the complainant's vulval and perianal swabs. If the assailant's DNA profile is obtained, this can be used to support the allegation, although the precise interpretation will depend upon whether the complainant was subjected to other sexual acts that could account for the presence of the DNA (e.g. ejaculation). There are no published persistence data with regard to the maximum time during which it is possible to obtain the assailant's DNA pattern from the female genitalia following the act of cunnilingus or anilingus.

The Forensic Science Service has a presumptive test to identify blood but currently has no specific confirmatory test to distinguish between menstrual or traumatic blood. A retrospective survey carried out at the Metropolitan Police Forensic Science Laboratory found that nearly one-third of the vaginal swabs received from sexual assault complainants were bloodstained. It is therefore important that, whenever bleeding is noted during the medical examination, the forensic practitioner should communicate the possible source of the bleeding on the MEDX 1A form.

Following detection of a body fluid, DNA STR analysis may be undertaken in an attempt to identify the offender and to prove sexual contact. The current DNA recognition systems employed by the Forensic Science Service give greatly improved discrimination with improved sensitivity.[39] This is advantageous when dealing with small quantities of DNA, as are often observed in sexual assault cases. They are the technique of choice for profiles currently being entered and on to the National DNA Database in the UK[40-42] The system also contains all the Interpol and European Network of Forensic Science Institutes recommended European loci which provide points of comparisons for intelligence purposes outside the UK.[43-47]

A full profile should be obtained from vaginal swabs taken up to14 hours postcoitus. Partial profiles are more likely to be obtained between 24 and 48 hours postcoitus.[48] Female DNA profiles have been obtained on postcoital penile swabs up to 24 hours postcoitus.[49] It should be noted that there are currently no published persistence data regarding the possibility of obtaining a DNA STR profile from an assailant if no spermatozoa are present in the seminal fluid.

For very small amounts of DNA, low copy number profiling may be used in an attempt to obtain a STR profile. This handcrafted, highly sensitive procedure is an extension of the Forensic Science Service's SGM Plus® (Applied Biosystems, Foster City, CA, USA) PCR amplification technique, which has lead to an increase in sample types being amenable to DNA testing. This, in turn, can provide valuable intelligence to the police.[50]

There are no published data with regard to the persistence of body fluids other than saliva and the time that DNA analysis is successful on unwashed skin. Inevitably, the amount of recoverable material will diminish with time. DNA profiles have been recovered from saliva deposited on skin up to 48 hours after deposition on cadavers.[51] Several studies have reported that that the biting of female breasts occurs in 7–19% of sexual offences,[52,53] so it is important to ask the complainant whether biting or sucking of the breasts occurred during the sexual assault.

The Forensic Science Service offers additional DNA intelligence products that may add to an investigation where the description of the offender is unknown by the complainant. Inferring ethnic origin by means of the STR profile obtained from a crime stain is one method.[54] Red hair analysis is another test that is available and this test provides information on whether DNA recovered from a sample could have originated from an individual with naturally occurring red hair, including redheads who have greyed due to the ageing process. The technique can be applied to extracts generated from SGM Plus® analysis and has been developed using a minisequencing protocol.[55]

Lubricant trace evidence may supplement biological evidence or may be the primary physical evidence where biological evidence is unavailable. Swabs taken from the genitalia may therefore be required to be examined for lubricants, in particular condom lubricant. Condom lubricant examination has been considered previously where either party says that a condom was used and also in cases where a complainant is attacked from the rear or where recollection of events is uncertain, such as in drug-facilitated sexual assault.

The identification of lubricant can, in some cases, provide confirmatory evidence of recent penetration of an intimate body orifice. The requirement to test for lubricant is often overlooked if the complainant does not mention that something was used during the assault. For this reason, two swabs are usually required when sampling the genitalia. There are four basic types of lubricant:

- silicone-based, found in most condoms
- polyethylene glycol (PEG)-based, found in few condoms
- water-based, e.g. KY Jelly® (Johnson&Johnson)
- oil-based.

A report published by the Forensic Science Service[56] found that the water-insoluble silicone lubricant persisted for at least 48 hours on the penis and at least 30 hours in the vagina. PEG had a poor persistence of around five hours. The Forensic Science Service has, for many years, been testing for the presence of condom lubricants on penile and vaginal swabs. The most commonly encountered condom lubricants are silicone-based oils, of which the most common is polydimethylsiloxane (PDMS; known commercially as Dimethicone®) or Simethicone®, polyethylene glycol (PEG) and aqueous formulations. Traces of PDMS have been identified from quality-assurance tests under taken on blank control swabs. A number of household products and medicinal preparations were also identified as containing PDMS. For this reason, PDMS testing has been withdrawn from casework while the problem is investigated (Bob Bramley, Chief Scientist, Priory House Birmingham Laboratory Forensic Science Service, personal communication, May 2004).

Methods of swabbing

At present, there is no internationally agreed method for obtaining samples from the female genital area. In the UK, best-practice guidelines were introduced by the tripartite Medical Examination Kit Working Party (consisting of representatives from the Association of Chief Police Officers, the Association of Police Surgeons and the Forensic Science Service), following the results obtained from research undertaken by Sweet et al.[57] These guidelines are included as Appendix 7.1 to this chapter.

The double-swab technique described by Sweet et al.[57] is the method recommended for recovering dried stains from skin, as it showed a higher percentage recovery of saliva from human skin. The first swab tip should be moistened using water from the ampoule provided in the module. Ensure maximum contact with the skin by rotating the swab, then use a second dry swab reapplied to the same area, ensuring that any moisture remaining is recovered. It should be noted that only minimal pressure should be applied to prevent exfoliation of the patient's own epithelial cells. Some protocols suggest that, where crusted material is visible, it should be scraped rather then swabbed.[58] The author knows of no evidence base to suggest this to be the more appropriate sample.

At the end of the use of the swab module, place an unopened swab, labelled as a control swab, in a separate, labelled tamper-evident bag.

Any sample collected using the swab module should be placed in a labelled, tamper-evident bag and frozen until transported to the forensic laboratory. Note that, where two swabs are taken from one site, they should be placed into one bag.

Alcohol and drug urine module

The purpose of this module is to collect a urine sample for qualitative toxicology analysis when drugs (drugs of abuse and medicinal) or alcohol have been consumed, or possibly administered prior to or during a sexual assault.

The length of time that alcohol, a drug or its metabolites remain detectable in urine is generally longer in urine than in a blood sample. The metabolites of some substances may be excreted for up to 168 hours in the urine. Gamma hydroxybutyrate (GHB), on the other hand, is only normally excreted for 6–12 hours in the urine, depending upon the dose.[59] For this reason, the urine specimen should be collected as soon as practically possible and can be taken prior to the forensic medical examination.

The current guideline issued by the Forensic Science Service is to collect a urine sample routinely in all sexual assault cases, from complainants and suspects, if the sexual assault is within four days of the forensic medical examination. If the allegation exceeds this time limit, the local forensic laboratory should be consulted on whether or not a urine sample is required for toxicology analysis.

The sample is collected by the complainant herself and does not have to be witnessed. The urine should be passed into the plastic collection beaker. Complainants should be advised not to dispose of any tampons, towels or panty liners that they may be wearing and should not be asked to collect toilet tissue.

Twenty ml urine is then decanted into the urine container (fill to the line and do not exceed), which has a white coating of sodium fluoride to prevent fermentation of the sample. Secure the screw cap and invert several times to mix with the preservative. Place into a labelled, tamper evident bag and refrigerate until transported to the forensic laboratory.

Alcohol and drug blood module

This module is for a blood sample for quantitative toxicology analysis when drugs (drugs of abuse and medicinal) or alcohol have been consumed, or possibly administered prior to or during a sexual assault. A blood sample for analysis of drugs and alcohol should be requested routinely from complainants and suspects in all sexual assault cases where the incident has occurred within four days of the forensic medical examination. This routine request for both blood and urine is relevant, even in those who deny alcohol or drug use in relation to the offence, because a negative result may be relevant to a subsequent trial.

Ten ml of venous blood is required. The blood should be obtained from a vein in the antecubital fossa or another accessible vein in the arm or hand. If it is not possible to obtain the sample of blood from the arm or hand, the venepuncture should be aborted and the police advised that they will have to rely on urine alone for forensic analysis.

The blood is placed into the screw-topped container (note that the rubber septum should be removed prior to the sample being injected into the bottle) and then insert the septum before securing the screw cap. The bottle contains a white coating of sodium fluoride and potassium oxalate to prevent fermentation and coagulation of the sample. Invert the sample several times to mix with the preservative. Place the blood container inside the secure container with the extra packing material provided to protect the bottle and then into a labelled tamper-evident bag. Refrigerate until transported to the forensic laboratory.

If solvent abuse is suspected then a portion of blood must be collected in a separate RTA (Road Traffic Act) vial (this is a dedicated container with a septum and aluminium cap and is not provided in the medical examination kit). This vial should not filled more than half full. Place into a labelled tamper-evident bag and refrigerate until transported to the forensic laboratory.

The Forensic Science Service routinely analyses known blood and urine samples containing low levels of drugs associated with drug-facilitated sexual assault; that is, levels expected when the drug is on the verge of disappearing from the body. Therefore, it is possible to be 100% certain that, had such a drug been present, it would have been detected by the analytical methods currently employed if the samples were taken within two to four days of the offence occurring.

The results of many Forensic Science Service cases tested to date show that genuine instances where a person has been given a sedative drug unknowingly are very few. By far the most common, significant finding is the presence of large amounts of alcohol in the majority of cases.[60] Alcohol is also readily available and mostly consumed voluntarily by complainants in these types of offences.

DNA 2 buccal kit

In order to obtain a reference DNA sample from a complainant or suspect of a sexual assault allegation easily, a DNA buccal kit is used. This is a non-intrusive sample which is easy to obtain and does not require a forensic medical examiner to collect. If a sample is recovered for evidential court purposes from a suspect, i.e. to prove or disprove involvement in the sexual offence under investigation, the DNA 2 kit can be used for this purpose. The suspect's profile can be loaded into the National DNA Database.

The paperwork provided with the kit is completed according to the complainant's status. Note that a complainant's reference sample is only ever taken for elimination purposes and is never loaded into the database.

The person taking the sample should wear the gloves provided throughout the whole procedure and avoid talking, coughing, etc., over the sample. Take one of the two mouth swabs provided and peel the polythene cover to reveal the swab. Taking care to hold the stem end, place the swab end into the donor's mouth and scrape the swab firmly against the inside of the cheek five or six times. Open one of the flip-top sample containers; the swab should then be ejected into the sample container by pressing the stem end towards the swab. Once the sample is placed inside the container tube the top must be closed. The whole procedure should then be repeated using the second mouth swab and tube on the other inner cheek. Both containers should then be placed into the small tamper-evident bag provided and sealed. Complete the DNA 2 sample and place this with the sealed samples into the large tamper-evident bag. Do not remove the spare bar codes. Freeze the sample until transported to the forensic laboratory.

If, at any time during the sampling process, the swab is dropped or comes into contact with any other surface, the procedure should stop and the sampling kit disposed of. The samples must then be taken again using a new DNA sampling kit.

Problems associated with collecting forensic samples

This part of the chapter highlights the problems associated with collecting forensic samples using the medical examination kit and focuses on the realities of obtaining evidence from these samples.

Basic scientific principles for the collection and analysis of forensic samples

It has been observed that, even though a national standard has been recommended by the National Medical Examination Kit Working Party, a number of different kits are being used by law enforcement agencies throughout the UK. This has led to inconsistency in evidence collection, with different kits collecting different amounts of evidence. In some cases, the amount of samples and containers falls short of what is actually required to complete a full forensic examination, particularly where a number of skin swabs are collected. In these situations, a further kit has to be used to achieve what is required. This is not cost effective and is one of the reasons for the development of an audit group whose focus is the continuous assessment of use of the medical examination kit.

The audit group regularly receives suggestions for improvements from forensic medical examiners, police officers, forensic scientists and complainants of sexual assault. The purpose of this group is to strive for continuous improvement in the way that evidence is collected from adult and child complainants and from suspects involved in serious sexual assaults. The kit contents need to evolve to meet the needs of the complainant and any changing requirements caused by technological progress. This should also be paralleled by changes in storage of kit samples. Improvements will only occur if dialogue between police, forensic medical examiners and scientists is continuing.

It is also essential to collect, analyse and publish data on the nature of the sexual assaults observed in the UK and of the medical findings in these cases, which, in turn, will inform future forensic strategy for such investigations. Developments for the future may involve the use of dedicated kits.[61] It is important that the recommended kit provides the necessary tools for the appropriate collection of evidence in a way in that is respectful to the patient.

The Forensic Science Service is currently investing time and resources into investigating the wider impacts of minimum scientific standards. For example, all evidence recovery products and kits supplied by the Service used for sampling biological material for DNA profiling purposes undergo stringent quality control tests. A strict quality control testing programme has been developed in order to ensure that no detectable levels of DNA are present on the kit components supplied to police forces. It is recognised that if quality control validation is not available there may be a violation of scientific principles.[62,63]

Packaging and continuity

The adhesive tamper-evident seal on the exhibit bags provided in all the modules is water based and therefore dehydration over a period of time could result in the seal being less effective. The manufacturer can only offer a seal guarantee up to the printed expiry date on the bag, so the date on the bag should be observed before sealing the sample. The Forensic Science Service has dealt with several cases where evidence was disputed in Court because of expired tamper-evident bags being used.[64]

Storage of samples

Outside the UK, cardboard boxes are used for the drying and storage of swabs collected during sexual assault examinations.[65] The author has no information about whether air-dried samples have any benefit over frozen samples. Both methods present problems with regard to storage space in the long term.

Concerns with specific modules

Medical examination documentation module

The pro formas in this module are a useful tool as they provide the capability of collating data to inform forensic strategy surrounding the relevance of specimens collected, effects of packaging and storage of samples and persistence data.

A copy of the pro formas should be forwarded to the forensic laboratory with any samples submitted in a sexual assault case. In practice, this paperwork is only received in 60% of cases.

The question really is who is best placed to record and collate the data? The forensic laboratory could retrieve information from the pro formas and compare this against forensic results obtained from samples in the case. The collective data could then be made available to the law enforcement agencies and other disciplines involved in the investigation of sexual assault offences. The reality is that this would be a timely process and without financial support is not something the Forensic Science Service has routinely offered to date. A pilot scheme has just been developed to include this type of monitoring for a small number of police forces and the results of the feasibility study will be available in June 2004.[66]

When recording information necessary to perform the medical and evidentiary examination, the practitioner must be careful not to include any subjective opinions or conclusions as to whether a crime occurred. The indiscriminate use of wording such as "semen is present" may prejudice future legal proceedings, particularly where the forensic laboratory does not identify semen on swabs forwarded to them for examination.

Disposable clothing module

Some law enforcement agencies request that the paper pants are put on by the complainant after the medical examination and worn home. A visit is then made to the complainant within a few hours of the medical examination so that the disposable pants can be retrieved. The thought behind this is that further drainage of body fluid may occur, which can be subsequently collected. There is no evidence base to indicate this is a worthwhile exercise and, in addition to the intimate swabs collected during a medical examination, any clothing worn at the time of the offence that was in close contact with the genitalia would be more relevant for examination. This exercise only serves to provide the patient with additional and unnecessary trauma.

Body outline diagram module

Although the diagrams are the property of the practitioner, on occasion it will be useful to provide relevant copies to the forensic laboratory as an *aide mémoire*; for example, if the patient was bitten there would be a possibility that saliva was deposited on the patient's body or clothing. Without precise information of where the bite occurred it is a time-consuming examination for the scientist to search for the presence of saliva, particularly on the clothing.

Mouth collection module

There is no current worldwide consensus as to which is the best sampling method where oral–penile contact is alleged. Samples other than those included in this medical examination kit include the use of interdental toothbrushes,[67,68] gauze pads, chewing gum[69] or filter paper,[70] none of which, to the author's knowledge, have extended the persistence time limits for detecting spermatozoa in the oral cavity. Chewing gum, while a logical sample to stimulate the production of saliva, which is often problematic in the traumatised patient, presents the forensic laboratory with problems in terms of the extraction of cellular material and is not used in the UK.

There are no published data regarding the persistence of the complainant's DNA STR profile from samples from the assailant's oral cavity or lips following an allegation of cunnilingus or anilingus. Apart from anecdotal information from forensic casework results of face swabs there is little published on the persistence of DNA STR profiles on lip swabs where kissing has occurred. The work of Banaschak et al.[71] obtained mixed DNA STR profiles in five samples obtained from five couples who had kissed for two minutes. However, in all cases, the kissing partner's DNA STR pattern was only identifiable immediately after kissing and no mixed profiles were identified when the volunteers were retested again after five minutes. In a casework situation, the kissing would be unlikely to persist for very long and samples would not be collected within minutes of an offence occurring. It is therefore important that the mouth swab from the early evidence kit is used as soon as is practicably possible in stranger assaults if the complainant alleges kissing by the assailant.

Hair collection module

Studies vary on how often pubic hair transfer occurs between complainant and suspect.[72–74] It should be noted that the Forensic Science Service rarely carries out hair comparisons in sexual assault cases. The fact that recovered hairs from the complainant and suspect can be of some evidential value in the prosecution of a serious sexual assault is not disputed. The issue is whether that value justifies the collection of control samples at the time of the medical examination. In the rare circumstances that it should become necessary to perform comparison microscopy, a control sample from the complainant can be obtained later.[75]

There is a division of opinion among professionals as to the method of collecting control hair samples by combing, cutting or pulling.[58,75–78] It must be borne in mind that, although the complainant is indeed considered as a crime scene, a humane approach to the collection of forensic samples must be paramount in the investigation.

Fingernail sample collection module

Many law enforcement agencies outside the UK collect samples from fingernails using small pointed swabs. It could be argued that this is a better method of retrieval than scraping, particularly where nails are long.[79] This method of sampling is currently being explored by the Forensic Science Service and will be included in the medical examination kit if the yield of recovered material is significant. The procedure of scraping or swabbing if clippings are not an option will be at the discretion of the practitioner. The recovery of DNA matching the complainant from an offender's fingernails who is not previously known to them may be of strong evidential value if contact is denied. However the testing of all ten fingernails in an endeavour to recover foreign DNA can be a significant drain on laboratory resources. The examination of this sample needs to be weighed up against the likelihood of recovering a useful result.[80] Neville states that 38% of individuals have DNA from someone other than themselves under their fingernails and that DNA is recovered from the majority of fingernails examined. The most likely outcome is that the DNA recovered will match the donor of the nails, especially if the nails show evidence of blood staining.

Swab module

The focus on particular STR loci to form a core system for creating a national DNA database does mean that there may be implications for the future of forensic science intelligence if it is decided to move to a new genetic system. Currently, the only contender is single nucleotide polymorphism (SNP) analysis. For this to be a realistic alternative, advantages in cost and ease of use will have to be demonstrated.

The Forensic Science Service is currently researching the use of FISH, with a Y chromosome-specific DNA probe, to identify small amounts of male epithelial cells that can subsequently be isolated allowing STR DNA profiling to be carried out on the recovered material.[81-83] This will be useful in cases where the offender is suspected of being oligospermic or aspermic, or where minimal amounts of male epithelial cells may be deposited, for instance on skin swabs, hand swabs of a suspect who has performed digital penetration and hand swabs from a complainant who alleges masturbation of the suspect's penis.[84] Dziegelewski et al.[85] have reported Y chromosome intact cells being recovered on postcoital vaginal swabs seven days later. In addition, Y chromosome-positive cells have been identified from vaginal swabs taken immediately after intercourse where no ejaculation has occurred.[85]

When reporting findings or providing expert evidence, the scientist must be able to rely on the forensic practitioner to obtain the swab samples in a manner that will refute any later suggestions by the defence that significant quantities of spermatozoa, which were only deposited on the outside, could have accidentally been transferred to the inside during the medical examination.[34] There has been no research to support or refute this hypothesis to date but the Forensic Science Service research and development group has been asked to consider a research proposal looking at this potential problem.[86]

Many guidelines outside the UK call for immediate wet-mount examinations from the swabbing of an orifice at the time of the medical examination, in an attempt to identify motile spermatozoa and provide the investigator with some information early on in the process. Motile sperm have been observed up to eight hours postcoitus on wet-mount slides. It has been demonstrated that searching of the native preparation often yields a false positive result and it is not considered good practice.[87,88] It is therefore recommended that the identification of spermatozoa be left to forensic experts. At the laboratory, time can be afforded with regard to specialist swab extraction, staining procedures and high-resolution microscopy in order to facilitate identification.

Outside the UK, in addition to the swabs indicated for collection from a female complainant, further samples are employed in the form of aspiration of any pools of fluid in the high vagina or placing 2–10 ml saline or sterile water in the vagina and then aspirating the washings.[89,90] However, aspirates should not be necessary if paired swabs are used to sample the vagina in the manner described in the first part of this chapter. Furthermore, there are no data to confirm that vaginal washings retrieve spermatozoa more effectively or at longer times after intercourse than vaginal swabs.

With the advent of DNA LCN (low copy number) analysis and its application in serious crime cases, it is important that practitioners become more intuitive in their approach to sampling. For example, in an assault carried out by a stranger, consideration should be given to sampling areas of the body that may have visible marks from where the complainant may have been touched by the offender. A DNA LCN profile has been obtained from grip marks on a female complainant's arms sampled 40 minutes after she was attacked by a stranger.[91] The problem with this type of sampling is that there is still considerable lack of understanding about issues of transfer and persistence and common sense would dictate that 'speculative' swabbing of skin should not be carried out unless visible marks or injuries are present. The Forensic Science Service research and development unit is considering further research in this area.

The disadvantage with the sensitivity of the DNA STR analysis employed by the Forensic Science Service, particularly where low copy number analysis is carried out, is that practitioners must take all possible steps to ensure that the samples they obtain are not contaminated by their own cellular material. To this end, the practitioner should always wear gloves when obtaining the samples. The practitioner must also avoid talking, coughing or sneezing over any sample; if this is a possibility then a disposable facemask should be worn and the reason explained to the complainant.

A striking paucity of literature exists pertaining to the examination of the penis of an alleged assailant for potential evidence indicative of sexual assault. In reality, this is because, even if the offender is known to the complainant, he is often examined too long after the offence for intimate samples collected from a medical examination to yield a positive, significant result.

In terms of lubricant analysis on swabs, practitioners should be aware that silicone is also found in numerous other products that may be applied to the body, e.g. skin care and bath products. PEG is found in ointments and suppositories. It is therefore important that the practitioner ask the complainant if anything has been applied to the genitalia and this should be recorded on the MEDX B form for the scientist's reference. If such a product has been used it will be necessary to check what lubricant it contains, if any. This may alter the scientist's interpretation of any findings. Dusting agents may also be detected, in the form of starch grains and *Lycopodium* spores, and can be used to corroborate the finding of condom lubricant. The practitioner must therefore prevent contamination by wearing non-powdered gloves at all times. *Lycopodium* spores are not used by the main UK manufacturers, because of potential health hazards, including asthma.[92,93]

The forensic laboratory will not routinely test for condom lubricant on an offender's penile swabs, as a defence may be that a condom was used shortly before or subsequent to the time of the alleged assault. However, such analysis may still be relevant in establishing the credibility of the prosecution and defence propositions. The detection of any condom lubricants on vaginal swabs from casework in reality yields few positive results. The general advice currently given by the Forensic Science Service is that if vaginal swabs are taken more than six hours and anal swabs more than eight hours following intercourse there is little chance of detecting any condom lubricants, even if it is known that one was used.[94]

KY jelly® and other lubricants should be avoided on specula and proctoscopes, as swabs contaminated by such lubricants yield significantly less DNA and lubricants may have been used in the incident. If the practitioner decides for clinical reasons to use KY Jelly® then care should be taken not to contaminate the swab samples. The KY Jelly® used must be a single-sachet application and the used sachet should be submitted in a separate labelled, tamper-evident bag as a reference in case lubricant analysis is required.

Alcohol and drug urine collection module

Forensic samples are often taken too late to yield positive results. Hence, many police forces have taken the initiative to use the drug and alcohol urine and mouth collection modules in the medical examination kit for the collection of early evidence. It has, however, been observed that the distribution of medical examination kits is often restricted to rape examination suites and the availability of the modules is too restricted. Thus, a separate, dedicated early evidence kit has been developed to allow quick access to all potential users. The kit was developed by The Forensic Science Service together with the Metropolitan Police. As a result of the kit being highlighted as good practice by the HMIC/CPS(I) report on the Joint Inspection into the Investigation and Prosecution of Cases Involving Allegations of Rape, published in April 2002,[95] the Forensic Science Service is now offering the kit to all police forces in the UK. The early evidence kit provides the first-response officer with the necessary equipment and instructions to collect a urine and mouth swab as soon as possible after a serious sexual assault has been reported. It is of particular benefit where there may be a time delay before a medical examination can take place.[96]

The greatest problem in drug-facilitated sexual assault is that complainants often do not report the incident in a timely manner because of amnesia and doubt about what may have happened. Some protocols do not advocate the routine procedure of collecting blood and urine for toxicology screening because of this time delay. The Texas protocol[58] suggests this should only be undertaken if the complainant or another witness states that the complainant was involuntarily drugged by an assailant and or it is the opinion of the practitioner that the complainant's medical condition appears to warrant toxicological screening for optimal care.

New methods of analysis may enable substances to be detected for longer periods, which is particularly important in allegations of drug-facilitated sexual assault, where the report is often delayed for several days.[97-99] Hair would appear to be a logical specimen choice where a delay in reporting occurs. Currently there are few laboratories that analyse hair for drugs and the methods employed were originally designed to detect chronic drug use and not for single dose analysis.[100-102] It should be noted, therefore, that hair specimens are not conducive to comprehensive drug screens and sample can be quickly consumed in testing for a few drugs. Most importantly, hair cannot be used to screen for the most commonly encountered drug in drug-facilitated sexual assault – alcohol. Therefore, the Forensic Science Service is currently not offering toxicological analysis of hair.

It is important that complainants who report this type of offence four or more days after it happened are informed about the realities of toxicological testing and that, where a negative result is obtained from blood or urine, an explanation is provided about the meaning of such a result.

In many cases reported, because of the time delay, there are no findings in the blood or urine samples tested by the Forensic Science Service.

Alcohol and drug blood collection module

The current collection system was introduced as an interim measure while the Forensic Science Service sourced a fit-for-purpose forensic vacuum container system. Once a suitable replacement has been identified this module will be updated.

DNA 2 kit

The complainant should refrain from smoking, eating or drinking for 20 minutes before the samples are taken, as this may affect the chances of buccal cell harvesting, which, in turn, may reduce the chance of obtaining a DNA profile. In cases involving oral sex between persons of the same gender, an additional buccal sample may be required several days later. The laboratory will advise if this is a requirement.

Summary

In summary, this chapter has given an overview of the current practices used in the UK when taking forensic samples from sexual assault adult complainants and suspects. The practices have only come about by determination to improve the care of women complainants by those dealing with them. Thus, the evidence obtained from both the medical and scientific sources is a good as it can currently be.

Complainants of sexual assault who perceive that their care was organised and respectful are more likely to return for follow-up counselling and treatment and, importantly, are more likely to encourage others to report offences.

References

1. Kevin Sullivan, Priory House, Birmingham Laboratory, Forensic Science Service. Personal communication (2002).
2. Keating SM, Allard JE. What's in a name? Medical samples and scientific evidence in sexual assaults. *Med Sci Law* 1994;34:187–201.
3. Negrusz A, Gaensslen RE. Toxicological Investigations in Drug-Facilitated Sexual Assault. *Problems of Forensic Sciences* 2000;41:7–18.
4. Keating SM. The Laboratory's approach to sexual assault cases. Part 1: Sources of information and acts of intercourse. *J Forensic Sci Soc* 1988;28:35–47.
5. Clark MDB. Metropolitan Police Laboratory examination kit for sexual offences. *The Police Surgeon* 1979;15:447–52.
6. Association of Police Surgeons. *After Care Leaflet in Sexual Offences Kit.* Glasgow; APS; 2001.
7. Association of Chief Police Officers. *What Happens Now?* London: ACPO; 2001.
8. Medley S, Metropolitan Police Service. Personal communication, 2002.
9. Allard JE. The collection of data from findings in cases of sexual assault and the significance of spermatozoa on vaginal, anal and oral swabs. *Sci Justice* 1997;37:99–108.
10. Enos WF, Beyer JC. Spermatozoa in the anal canal and rectum and in the oral cavity of female rape victims. *J Forensic Sci Soc* 1978;23:231–3.

11. King P, Donnelly A, Silenieks E, Flinders University, Adelaide. Unpublished data, 2002.
12. Enos WF, Beyer JC. The importance of examining skin and hair for semen in sexual assault cases. *J Forensic Sci Soc* 1981;26:605–7.
13. Sansom P, London Laboratory, Forensic Science Service. Personal communication, 2002.
14. Young WW, Bracken AC, Goddard MA, Matheson S. Sexual assault: review of a national model protocol for forensic and medical evaluation. New Hampshire Sexual Assault Medical Examination Protocol Project Committee. *Obstet Gynecol* 1992;80:878–83.
15. Prahlow JA, Lantz PE, Cox-Jones K, Rao PN, Pettenati MJ. Gender identification of human hair using fluorescence in situ hybridisation. *J Forensic Sci* 1996;41:1035–7.
16. Higuchi R, Von Beroldingen CH, Sensabaugh GF, Erlich HA. DNA from single hairs. *Nature* 1988;332:543–6.
17. Tully G, Morley JM, Bark JE. Forensic analysis of mitochondrial DNA: application of multiple solid-phase-fluorescent minisequencing to high throughput analysis. Proceedings of the 2nd European Symposium on Human Identification, Innsbruck, June 1998. p. 92–6.
18. Morley JM, Bark JE, Evans CE, Perry JG, Hewitt CA, Tully G. Validation of mitochondrial DNA minisequencing for forensic casework. *Int J Legal Med* 1999;112:241–8.
19. Pugh RK, Huntingdon Laboratory Forensic Science Service. Personal communication, 2002.
20. Salter MT, Cook R. Transfer of fibres to head hair, their persistence and retrieval. *Forensic Sci Int* 1996;81:211–21.
21. Oz C, Zamir A. An evaluation of the relevance of routine DNA typing of fingernail clippings for forensic casework. *J Forensic Sci* 2000;45:158–60.
22. Mustoe S, London Laboratory Forensic Science Service. Personal communication, 2002.
23. Moore E, Chorley Laboratory Forensic Science Service. Personal communication, 1998.
24. Harris E, London Laboratory Forensic Science Service. Personal communication, 1998.
25. Wallin JM, Buoncristiani MR, Lazaruk KD, Fildes N, Holt CL, Walsh PS. TWGDAM validation of the AmpFLSTR™ Blue PCR amplification kit for forensic casework analysis. *J Forensic Sci* 1998;43:854–70.
26. Lederer T, Seidl S, Graham B, Betz P. A new pentaplex PCR system for forensic casework analysis. *Int J Legal Med* 2000;114:87–92.
27. Lederer T, Betz P, Seidl S. DNA analysis of fingernail debris using different multiplex systems: a case report. *Int J Legal Med* 2001;114:263–6.
28. Vintiner SK, Harbinson SA, Petricevic SF, Forensic Biology Group, Institute of Environmental Science and Research, Auckland, New Zealand. Unpublished data.
29. Bates M, Wetherby Laboratory Forensic Science Service. Personal communication, 2002.
30. Thomas F, Baert H. A new means of identification of the human being: the longitudinal striation of the nails. *Med Sci Law* 1965;5:39–40.
31. Medley S, Metropolitan Police Service. Personal communication, 2002.
32. Austin C, London Laboratory Forensic Science Service. Personal communication, 2002.
33. Sullivan K, Trident Court Birmingham Laboratory Forensic Science Service. Personal communication, 2002.
34. The Forensic Science Service. 2002. Qiagen. [http://128.1.18.1/html/qiagen/index.htm].
35. Keating SM, Allard JE. What's in a name? Medical samples and scientific evidence in sexual assaults. *Med Sci Law* 1994;34:187–201.
36. Keating SM. The laboratory's approach to sexual assault cases. Part 2. Demonstration of the possible offender. *J Forensic Sci Soc* 1988;28:99–110.
37. Florence A. Du sperme et des taches de sperme en medecine legale. *Arch d'Anthropol Criminelle d Criminolo Psychol Normale Pathol* 1896;11:146–65.
38. Bob Bramley, Chief Scientist, Priory House Birmingham Laboratory Forensic Science Service. Personal communication, 2002.

39. Cotton EA, Allsop RF, Guest JL, Frazier RRE, Koumi P, Callow IP, *et al. Forensic Sci Int* 2000;112:151–61.
40. Foreman LA, Evett IW. Statistical analyses to support forensic interpretation for a new ten-locus STR profiling system. *Int J legal Med* 2001;114:147–55.
41. Gill P. Role of short tandem repeat DNA in forensic casework in the UK-past, present and future perspectives. *Biotechniques* 2002;32:366–72.
42. Werrett DJ. Forensics. The national DNA database. *Forensic Sci Int* 1997;88:33–42.
43. Hoyle R. The FBI's national DNA database. *Nat Biotechnol* 1998;16:987.
44. Gill P, Sparkes, Fereday L, Werrett DJ. Report of the European Network of Forensic Science Institutes (ENSFL): formulation and testing of principles to evaluate STR multiplexes. *Forensic Sci Int* 2000;108:1–29.
45. Bar W, Brinkmann B, Budowle B, Carracedo A, Gill P, Lincoln P, *et al.* DNA recommendations. Further report of the DNA Commission of the ISFH regarding the use of short tandem repeat systems. International Society for Forensic Haemogenetics. *Int J Legal Med* 1997;110:175–6.
46. Olaisen B, Bar W, Brinkmann B, Budowle B, Carracedo Gill P, *et al.* DNA recommendations 1997 of the International Society for Forensic Genetics. *Vox Sang* 1998;74:61–3.
47. Leriche A, Vanek D, Schmitter H, Schleenbecker U, Woller J, Montagna P, *et al.* Final report of the Interpol Working Party on DNA Profiling. Proceedings from the 2nd European Symposium on Human Identification, 1998. Madison, WI: Promega Corporation [www.promega.com/geneticidproc/eursymp2proc/13.pdf]. Accessed 31 July 2003.
48. Elliott K, Trident Court Birmingham Laboratory Forensic Science Service. Success rates from postcoital swabs. Unpublished data, 2002.
49. Stephen JC, Collins KA, Pettenati MJ, Fitts M. Isolation and identification of female DNA on postcoital penile swabs. *Am J Forensic Med Pathol* 2000;21:97–100.
50. The Forensic Science Service. Low Copy Number DNA Profiling. [http://128.1.18.1/html/corpcomm/hotnews/low_copy.htm].
51. Sweet D, Lorente JA, Valenzuela A, Lorente M, Villanueva E. PCR based DNA typing of saliva stains recovered from human skin. *J Forensic Sci* 1997;42:447–51.
52. Vale GL, Noguchi TT. Anatomical distribution of human bite marks in a series of 67 cases. *J Forensic Sci Soc* 1983;28:61–9.
53. Wright R, West DJ. Rape – a comparison of group offences and lone assaults. *Med Sci Law* 1981;21:25–30.
54. Lowe AL, Urquhart A, Foreman LA, Evett IW. Inferring ethnic origin by means of an STR profile. *Forensic Sci Int* 2001;119:17–22.
55. Shadwell J, Trident Court Birmingham Laboratory Forensic Science Service. Personal communication, 2002.
56. Thompson P, Chorley Laboratory Forensic Science Service. Forensic analysis of condom components. Unpublished data, 2001.
57. Sweet D, Lorente M, Lorente JA, Valenzuela A, Villanueva E. An improved method to recover saliva from human skin: The double swab technique. *J Forensic Sci* 1997;42:320–2.
58. Office of the Attorney General, Sexual Assault Prevention and Crisis Services Program. Texas Evidence Collection Protocol. 1998. [www.oag.state.tx.us/AG_Publications/pdfs/evidence_collection.pdf].
59. Jansen K. Date rape drugs. *Bull Int Assoc Forensic Toxicol* 1998;28:18–20.
60. Scenesafe Evidence Recovery Systems. K106 Early Evidence Kit. 2002. [www.fss.org.uk].
61. Pennsylvania State Nurses Association. Choosing the best sexual assault forensic exam kit. PA Coalition Against Rape. [http://www.psna.org/Practice/examkits.htm]. Accessed 31 July 2003.
62. Gill P, Trident Court Birmingham Laboratory Forensic Science Service. Personal communication, 2002.
63. Jheinga Bimal, Norfolk House, Birmingham Forensic Science Service. Personal communication, 2002.
64. Connolly Y, Chorley Laboratory Forensic Science Service. Personal communication, 2002.
65. Hochmeister M, Rudin O, Meier R, Peccioli M, Borer U, Eisenberg A, *et al.* A foldable

cardboard box for drying and storage of biological evidence collected on cotton swabs. *Arch Kriminol* 1997;200:113–20.

66. McCrossan S, Trident Court Laboratory, Birmingham Forensic Science Service. New ways of working. Personal communication, 2002.

67. London Laboratory Forensic Science Service Forensic Scientists. Personal communications, 1998.

68. Rogers D, Association of Forensic Physicians. Personal communication.

69. Lind W, Carlson D. Recovery of semen from chewing gum in an oral sexual assault. *Journal of Forensic Identification* 1995;45:280–2.

70. Hampton HL. Care of the woman who has been raped. *N Engl J Med* 1995;332:234–7.

71. Banaschak S, Moller K, Pfeiffer H. Potential DNA mixtures introduced through kissing. *Int J Legal Med* 19987;111:284–5.

72. Mann MJ. Hair transfers in sexual assault: a six year case study. *J Forensic Sci Soc* 1990;35:951–5.

73. Stone IC. Hair and its probative value as evidence. *Texas Bar J* 1982;45:275–9.

74. Riis R. Sexual assault combing evidence. Presented at the North West Association of Forensic Scientists, Jackson Hole, WY, 1990.

75. Roe G, London Laboratory Forensic Science Service. Personal communication, 2002.

76. Lewington F, Metropolitan Police Forensic Science Laboratory. Personal communication, 1994.

77. Enos WF, Beyer JC. The importance of examining skin and hair for semen in sexual assault cases. *J Forensic Sci Soc* 1981;26:605–7.

78. Immediate concerns after sexual assault. Aardvarc.org (Abuse, Rape And Domestic Violence Aid and Resource Collection). [http://aardvarc.org/rape/about/after.shtml]. Accessed 1 August 2003.

79. Scalise K, Department of Public Safety Regional Office, Garland Texas, USA. Personal communication, 2002.

80. Neville S, Institute of Clinical Pathology and Medical Research, Westmead Hospital, Sydney, Australia. Personal communication, 2002.

81. Collins KA, Rao PN, Hayworth R, Schnell S, Tap MP, Lantz PE, *et al.* Identification of sperm and non-sperm male cells in cervicovaginal smears using fluorescence *in situ* hybridisation. Applications in alleged sexual assault cases. *J Forensic Sci* 1994;39:1347–55.

82. Sibille I, Duverneuil C, Lorin de la Grandmaison G, Guerrouache K, Teissiere F, Durigon M, *et al.* Y-STR DNA amplification as biological evidence in sexually assaulted female victims with no cytological detection of spermatozoa. *Forensic Sci Int* 2002;125:212-16.

83. Rao PN, Collins KA, Geisinger KR, Parsons LH, Schnell S, Hayworth-Hodge R, *et al.* Identification of male epithelial cells in routine postcoital cervicovaginal smears using fluorescence *in situ* hybridisation. Application in sexual assault and molestation. *AM J Clin Pathol* 1995;104:32–5.

84. Elliott K. Trident Court Birmingham Laboratory Forensic Science Service. Personal communication, 2002.

85. Dziegelewski M, Simich JP, Rittenhouse-Olson K. Use of a Y chromosome probe as an aid in the forensic proof of sexual assault. *J Forensic Sci* 2002;47:601–4.

86. Allard J. London Laboratory Forensic Science Service. Personal communication, 2002.

87. Eungprabhanth V. Findings of the spermatozoa in the vagina related to elapsed time of coitus. *Z Rechtsmed* 1994;74:301–4.

88. Reade DJ. Early scientific investigations of sexual assault. *Police Surgeon* 1986(April):42–6.

89. Bradham GB. The establishment of treatment center for victims of rape. *J S C Med Assoc* 1981;77:283–6.

90. Robinson EG. Management of the rape victim. *CMAJ* 1976;115:520–3.

91. Burgess G, Wetherby Laboratory Forensic Science Service. Personal communication, 2002.

92. *Chemist and Druggist* 1995;243(5966):60.

93. McCrane WC, Delly JG. *The Particles Atlas.* Vol 3: p. 600, 702.

94. Condom Lubricants: A Summary. Chorley Laboratory Forensic Science Service. Unpublished data.

95. HM Crown Prosecution Service Inspectorate, HM Inspectorate of Constabulary. *A Report on the Joint Inspection into the Investigation and Prosecution of Cases Involving Allegations of Rape.* London: HMCPSI; April 2002. [www.homeoffice.gov.uk/hmic/CPSI_HMIC_Rape_Thematic.pdf]. Accessed 1 August 2003.

96. Newton MA, Jheinga B. User requirement for the K106 early evidence kit. Unpublished data.

97. Muller C, Vogt S, Goerke R, Kordon A, Weinmann W. Identification of selected psychopharmaceuticals and their metabolites in hair by LC/ESI-CID/MS and LC/MS/MS. *Forensic Sci Int* 2000;113:415–21.

98. Negrusz A, Moore CM, Kern JL, Janicak PG, Strong MJ, Levy NA. Quantitation of clonazepam and its major metabolite 7-aminoclonazepam in hair. *J Anal Toxicol* 2000;24:614–20.

99. Guterman L. Nailing the drug rapists. *New Scientist.* 1998;160:4.

100. Cirimele V, Kintz P, Staub C, Mangin P. Testing human hair for flunitrazepam and 7-amino-flunitrazepam by GC/MS-NCI. *Forensic Sci Int* 1997;84: 89–200.

101. Ropero-Miller JD, Goldberger BA, Cone EJ, Joseph RE. The disposition of cocaine and opiate analytes in hair and fingernails of humans following cocaine and codeine administration. *J Anal Toxicol* 2000;24:496–508.

102. Tsatsakis AM, Psillakis T, Paritsis N. Phenytoin concentration in head hair sections: a method to evaluate the history of drug use. *J Clin Psychopharmacol* 2000;20:560–73.

Appendix 7.1
Guidelines for sampling the female genitalia

Vaginal tract

Any external sanitary wear should be collected before sampling the genitalia. It is useful to record whether the item retrieved was in place during the sexual assault or whether the item collected has replaced something discarded since the incident.

The following swabs should be collected if vaginal intercourse has occurred within seven days or anal intercourse within three days of the medical examination. Note longer times for persistence are the exception rather than the rule.[1,2] The quantity of semen dedicated is also affected by the activity and posture of the complainant post assault which is why details such as washing and menstruation are recorded on form MEDX 1A.

If a lubricant or a condom was used, or suspected during the offence samples should be taken within 30 hours.

First sample

Sample the vulva rub using two dry swabs sequentially over the inner aspects of the labia majora, the labia minora and the vestibule. The swabs can initially be moistened with the ampoule of water if necessary. These swabs are labelled vulval swabs and numbered in the order taken.

Second sample

Sample the low vaginal tract taking two sequential swabs under direct vision. These swabs are labelled "low vaginal swabs" and numbered in the order taken.

Third sample

Sample the high vaginal tract, separate the labia and gently pass an appropriately sized transparent, disposable speculum two-thirds of the way into the vagina (if the speculum requires lubrication, use the ampoule of water provided). The speculum is then opened. If any foreign bodies are present, e.g. tampons or condoms, these should be removed and packaged separately. Then, two dry swabs are taken by sampling the vaginal tract beyond the end of the speculum, particularly the posterior fornix where any fluid may collect. The speculum is then removed unless an endocervical swab is required. These swabs are labelled "high vaginal swabs" and numbered in the order taken. It should be noted in certain circumstances, e.g. due to severe vaginal injuries, it may not be possible to pass a speculum. On these occasions, the swabs should be taken under direct vision, taking care to avoid contact with the vestibule and hymen. If no speculum is used this should be noted on form MEDX 1B. These swabs should be labelled 'vaginal swabs'.

The Forensic Science Service has had to examine the speculum for trace evidence in a number of cases to date. For this reason, it is now advocated as best practice that the speculum or a swab of the instrument should be retained, packaged in a separate labelled tamper-evident bag and stored frozen until transported to the laboratory. If the speculum is visibly wet on removal and swabbing is undertaken, several swabs may be recovered to retrieve material on the surface.

Final sample

In addition to the vaginal samples, a single endocervical swab should be collected if vaginal intercourse was more than 48 hours prior to the medical examination.[3-5] This sample is taken with the speculum still in place but manipulated to locate the cervix.

Rectum and anal canal

First sample

Sample the skin around the anus (approximate diameter to be sampled: 3 cm) using two sequential swabs moistened with the sterile water from the ampoule in the swab module.

Second sample

Pass a proctoscope (moistened with sterile water from the ampoule in the swab module) at least 3–4 cm into the anus, remove the obturator and sample the lower rectum using a single dry swab. The average anal canal is about 3 cm in the adult (range 1.4–3.8 cm in males and 1.0–3.2 cm in females). The mucosa of the upper anal canal is a deep purple colour, which readily distinguishes it from the red or pink mucosa of the lower rectum.

Third sample

Sample the anal canal using a single dry swab as the proctoscope is withdrawn. If it is not possible to pass a proctoscope, this should be noted on the MEDX 1B form and an attempt should be made to pass two dry swabs sequentially into the anus to sample the lower rectum and anal canal simultaneously. These swabs should be labelled "rectum/anal canal swabs".

References

1. Allard J. *The Facts of Life*. Contact No. 24. London: Forensic Science Service; 1996. p. 36–8. [Available from: info.services.enquiry.desk@fss.pnn.police.uk].
2. Davies A, Wilson E. The persistence of seminal constituents in the human vagina. *Forensic Sci* 1974;3:45–55.
3. Graves HCB, Sensabaugh GF, Blake ET. Postcoital detection of male-specific semen protein: application to the investigation of rape. *N Engl J Med* 1985;312:338–40.
4. Wilson EM. A comparison of the persistence of seminal constituents in the human vagina and cervix. *Police Surgeon* 1982;22:44–5.
5. Warner CG. *Rape and Sexual Assault Management and Intervention*. Germantown, MD: Aspen Systems Corp; 47–66.

Chapter 8

The genital examination

Deborah Rogers

Introduction

This chapter only relates to peripubertal and postpubertal females. The facts and dilemmas relating to prepubertal females are detailed in Chapter 16.

Aims and objectives

The aim of the genital examination is to document all relevant genital findings, in order to assist a court in its deliberations regarding the veracity of the allegation made by the complainant. It must be emphasised that in some cases there is no indication to examine the genital area; for example, if the complainant is adamant that fellatio (mouth to penis) was the only sexual act that took place during the assault.

Objectives of the genital examination

1. Identification and retrieval of any stains, secretions, fibres, hairs or particles that could be relevant to a police investigation (see Chapter 7).

2. Precise documentation of all injuries (fresh or healed) that might relate to the alleged incident.

3. Detection of any illnesses, diseases or signs of previous trauma that might affect the interpretation of the medical evidence.

Equipment

Complainants should be offered privacy while undressing (this can be achieved by means of a curtained area around the couch) and a gown and sheet or blanket to maintain their dignity during the genital and anal examination. Typically, the genital area is assessed with the complainant in the semilithotomy position and the perianal area is assessed with the complainant in the left lateral position on an examination couch.

Access to a cool light source and a magnifying lens is essential. Assessment of the vulva and hymen, particularly when fimbriated, may be facilitated by the gentle manipulation of the tissues with one or two swabs moistened with sterile water. In cases where the hymenal opening cannot initially be identified, 2–3 ml of warm sterile water should be dropped on to the hymen via a small syringe. This manoeuvre will often reveal the edge of the hymen. Complainants should be warned that the water might trickle on to the perineum.

Some practitioners recommend using a Foley catheter (size 8 or larger with a 50-ml capacity balloon) to aid visualisation of the hymen.[1] This is achieved by passing the catheter into the vagina until it is estimated that the balloon is in the mid-vagina. The balloon is then inflated with up to 50 ml of air (inflation should stop if the complainant experiences discomfort) and the catheter gently withdrawn until the inflated balloon reaches the introitus – the hymen will then be distended so that any tears or notches can be easily identified. In the acute setting, none of these interventions should be undertaken until the relevant forensic samples have been retrieved (see Chapter 7).

When the sampling or inspection of the vagina, anal canal or rectum is relevant, disposable specula and proctoscopes of various sizes must also be available.

Extent

The extent of the genital and anal examination will depend on the nature and timing of the allegation. In cases where the alleged assault is believed to have related to vaginal penetration, the vulval area should be carefully inspected for abnormalities and injuries after any necessary vulval swabs have been obtained. A precise note should be made of the configuration of the hymen. In particular, the presence of any notches and whether they are superficial (less than 50% the width of the hymenal rim) or deep (greater than 50% the width of the hymenal rim).

If the allegation relates to a vaginal penetrative act in the preceding 14 days, it may be necessary to sample the vagina and possibly the endocervical canal (see Chapter 7) and to inspect the vagina and cervix for injuries. This requires the use of a disposable speculum. Careful inspection of the vulva and hymen prior to using a speculum ensures that there can be no suggestion that any injuries were attributable to instrumentation.

In cases where the alleged assault is believed to have related to anal penetration, the perianal area should be carefully inspected for abnormalities and injuries after any necessary perianal swabs have been obtained. If the allegation relates to an anal penetrative act in the preceding three days, it will be necessary to sample the perianal area, anal canal and rectum (see Chapter 7). The anal canal and rectum are inspected for injuries via a proctoscope.

On occasion, a forensic practitioner may be asked to inspect the vulval area for signs of trauma many weeks or months following the alleged sexual act. This is only likely to be relevant if the complainant denies having experienced sexual acts other than the alleged assault. Similarly, inspection of the perianal area, anal canal and rectum many weeks or months after a single anal penetrative act is unlikely to yield positive findings unless the act caused significant tears to the skin or underlying muscle, as suggested by the symptoms described by the complainant subsequent to the assault.

Timing

The expediency of the genital examination should be determined on a case-by-case basis following consultation between an experienced forensic practitioner and the investigating officer. Table 6.1 in Chapter 6 (the persistence of spermatozoa) will inform this debate.

Clinical findings

To ensure consistency between practitioners with regard to obtaining forensic samples and describing injuries and abnormalities, it is imperative to use recognised terms to describe the location of the clinical findings and the site of sampling. Forensic scientists need to prioritise samples: if atypical terms are used to describe sites of sampling, the significance of the sample may be overlooked by a scientist who is not trained in anatomy.

It is traditional to refer to an imaginary clock face when describing the location of injuries or abnormalities on circumferential structures, e.g. the hymen and the perianal skin. The 12 o'clock position is always located immediately under the mons pubis and the six o'clock position is towards the coccyx, regardless of whether the complainant is in the prone or supine position (i.e. if the complainant is lying on her front, the 'clock' is upside down).

Vulva

The vulva is the collective term used to describe the external female genitalia (Figure 8.1). It incorporates the mons pubis, labia majora, labia minora, clitoris, clitoral hood and vestibule. The posterior margin of the vulva is bounded by the posterior fourchette: the site where the labia minora unite posteriorly. Most practitioners consider the posterior fourchette to be synonymous with the posterior labial commissure, although this term is frequently reserved for use in pre-pubertal females.[2] The urethra and the vagina open onto the vestibule.

The skin of the labia majora and the labia minora is keratinised squamous epithelium but only the outer aspects of the labia majora are hair-bearing. In the vestibule, the skin is nonkeratinised squamous epithelium with heavily glycogenated suprabasal cells; this appears shiny pink.[3]

The fossa navicularis is a relatively concave area of the vestibule that is bounded anteriorly by the vaginal opening, laterally by the labia minora and posteriorly by the posterior fourchette.

When the hypothalamic–pituitary–gonadal axis is reactivated in late childhood, the resultant secretion of sex hormones from the ovary causes

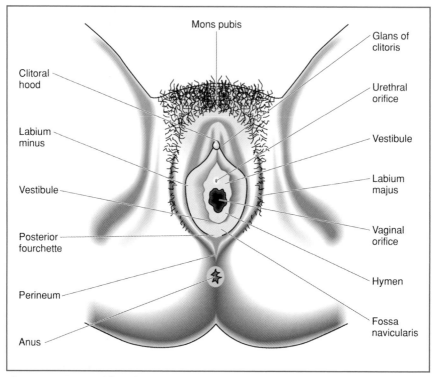

Figure 8.1 External female genitalia

the breasts and genitalia to alter in appearance. The most obvious change to the vulva is the development of pubic hair and this, together with the thelarche, is traditionally used to stage sexual development (Tanner staging; Figure 8.2). However, there are other important changes that occur to the vulva in terms of the enlargement of the mons, labia majora and labia minora, and the general thickening and increased elasticity of the genital skin.[4] In some females, the epithelium of the labia minora and vestibule becomes markedly prominent and folded. This is referred to as vulval papillomatosis or vestibular papillae and it may be mistaken for human papillomavirus infection.

Penile penetration of the vagina necessitates the penis passing between the labia minora and the hymenal opening. In most sexual positions, the apposition of the penis to the labia minora and posterior fourchette means that they may be stretched or rubbed as vaginal penetration is achieved. Lacerations, abrasions, bruises, petechiae, erythema and oedema have all been described on the vulva following consensual sexual activity, although some were only identified using a colposcope or following the application of toluidine blue.[5-8]

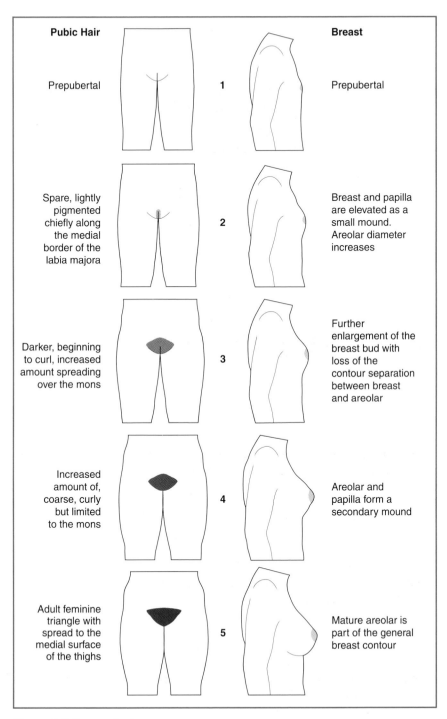

Pubic Hair | | **Breast**

Prepubertal — **1** — Prepubertal

Spare, lightly pigmented chiefly along the medial border of the labia majora — **2** — Breast and papilla are elevated as a small mound. Areolar diameter increases

Darker, beginning to curl, increased amount spreading over the mons — **3** — Further enlargement of the breast bud with loss of the contour separation between breast and areolar

Increased amount of, coarse, curly but limited to the mons — **4** — Areolar and papilla form a secondary mound

Adult feminine triangle with spread to the medial surface of the thighs — **5** — Mature areolar is part of the general breast contour

Figure 8.2 Tanner staging

All types of injuries have also been noted on the vulval area of complainants of sexual assault. Although most of the case series do not describe the precise site of the injury, in those that do the most common sites of injury were the posterior fourchette, the labia majora and minora, the hymen and the fossa navicularis.[5,9,10]

The vulval area heals well, usually leaving no or minimal scarring.[5,11] White midline structures in the fossa navicularis (linear vestibularis) have been described as a normal variant in females up to the age of ten years. It is not known whether they persist past puberty but it would be important to consider a linear vestibularis as part of the differential diagnosis for a possible scar in the fossa navicularis, particularly if it is not associated with surrounding neovascularisation.[12]

Hymen

The hymen is the tissue that partially or completely surrounds the opening of the vagina. Congenital absence of the hymen has never been recorded.[13] The hymen may be annular (completely encircling the vaginal opening), crescentic (present at the sides and posterior aspects of the vaginal opening but deficient at the suburethral area) or present only as interrupted tags or remnants (usually following childbirth). The latter may be referred to as carunculae hymenales.

There is usually a single opening in the hymen, which is referred to as the hymenal opening (this is synonymous with the vaginal introitus). Congenital variants of the hymenal morphology include two or more hymenal openings (respectively referred to as septate or cribriform hymens), a small anteriorly displaced opening (microperforate) and, occasionally, complete absence of an opening (imperforate hymen). The latter may be congenital or acquired.

Just as the vulva changes in appearance under the influence of the endogenous sex hormones, so does the hymen; it becomes thicker, elastic and more prominent. The oestrogenised hymen may protrude like a 'sleeve' or 'turtleneck collar' and may be described as 'redundant' whereby it folds on itself.[14] The edges may become 'scalloped' or 'fimbriated'.[14]

The terms 'acute tear' or 'acute laceration' are usually used to describe bleeding, full-thickness splits of the hymenal epithelium. Nonacute disruptions are variously described as healing or healed tears, healing or healed lacerations, transections, notches or clefts. However, the terms 'healed tear' and 'healed laceration' should only be used when the complainant has been previously examined and found to have a fresh tear or laceration at that site. Practitioners must be aware that superficial notches (less than 50% of the width of the hymenal rim) have been noted among nonabused prepubertal females[15] and, hence, such notches may have no significance among postpubertal females. However, it may not be possible to differentiate between a healed partial hymenal tear and a naturally occurring superficial notch.

For centuries, practitioners have been called upon to testify whether or not a female is a 'virgin'. The conclusion can have major significance in terms of a woman being murdered for having engaged in sexual activity before marriage or a man being found guilty of rape (and in some countries subjected to a death sentence). However, it has been recognised for many years that, contrary to popular belief, dogmatic statements regarding previous sexual activity of postpubertal females frequently cannot be made.[16] The postpubertal hymen is elastic and the current literature indicates that sexual activity does not necessarily cause it to tear. Emans *et al.*[17] found that, among 100 postmenarchal females (age range 9.5–28.0 years) who used tampons but who described themselves as sexually inactive, 11% only had complete transections of the hymen. If these figures are to be believed, this is evidence that, in the majority of postpubertal females, the hymen is elastic enough to accommodate a tampon without tearing.[17] There are no studies that specifically address how frequently the hymen tears following the first consensual penovaginal penetration. However, among complainants of sexual assault aged 14–19 years who stated that they were 'virgins' before the sexual assault, only 19% had acute hymenal tears.[18] Similarly, Biggs *et al.*[9] reported that, among 66 female complainants aged 15–64 years who denied sexual intercourse experience prior to the alleged assault, only 9.1% had hymenal tears. In addition, among the 100 females in the Emans *et al.*[17] study who stated that they were sexually active, 19% did not have a complete transection of the hymen.

Some practitioners feel that a digital assessment of the hymenal opening will reveal whether the woman had experienced penovaginal penetration. Although in a few women who have not experienced penovaginal penetration the hymen forms a tight ring inside the introitus, in others the hymen is so distensible that intercourse could have taken place.[16] Therefore, it is unwise for a forensic practitioner to state that a person has definitely had penovaginal intercourse.

In addition to lacerations (tears), bruises, abrasions, swelling and erythema have all been noted on the hymens of complainants of sexual assault examined within 72 hours of the assault.[3,18]

Bruises, abrasions, reddening and swelling of the hymen will completely disappear within a few days or weeks. Conversely, hymenal lacerations do not appear to reunite and thus will always remain apparent as partial or complete transections.[3]

Vagina

The vagina is the tubular structure that extends from the vestibule to the uterus. It should be noted that many lay people (including judges and barristers) erroneously use the term 'vagina' to describe the vulval area. This can lead to confusion with regard to the interpretation of a complainant's account of an incident and the medical evidence.

The lining of the prepubertal vagina is thin, appears red in colour, due to the visibility of the underlying blood vessels, and has relatively few rugae. The prepubertal cervix is flush with the vaginal vault and, hence, the fornices are not apparent. As the hypothalamic–pituitary axis becomes active in late childhood, the vagina lengthens from its late childhood length (7.0 cm to 8.5 cm) to its adult length of 10–12 cm, rugae develop and the cervix protrudes from the vault, forming the vaginal fornices.

Vaginal intercourse may cause minor or major injuries to the vagina. Fraser et al.[19] conducted two to three systematic vaginal inspections of 107 sexually active women aged 18–35 years with colposcopic magnification, to look for changes in the vaginal and cervical appearance that might be related to sexual intercourse. Changes in the vaginal surface appearance were observed in 56 (17.8%) of the 314 inspections. These were located at the introitus ($n = 6$), in the lower or middle thirds of the vagina ($n = 26$), on the forniceal surfaces of the cervix ($n = 8$), in the vaginal fornices ($n = 14$) and two showed generalised vaginal wall changes. The classification and frequency of the various changes are shown in Table 8.1. Some petechiae were produced during the assessment. Over 80% of the changes were difficult to detect with the naked eye and were only clearly seen with 6x–10x magnification using a colposcope. Sexual intercourse in the previous 24 hours was associated with an increased overall frequency of atypical changes.

Severe vaginal lacerations have been described in females aged 5–88 years. The majority occur in women of reproductive age. They occur in married and unmarried women and in women who have given birth to children as well as those who have not. Vaginal lacerations may be multiple or single. The majority occur at the top of the vagina but they may also occur along the sides. The length of the lacerations described in the literature varies from 2.0 cm to 8.5 cm.[20-22]

Table 8.1. Classification of changes in the vaginal and cervical appearance that might be related to sexual intercourse[19]

Classification	Frequency of occurrence (n)
Oedema	4
Erythema	9
Petechiae	30
Ecchymosis	2
Abrasion	5
Laceration	1
Micro-ulceration	3
Acetowhite	2

It is not known how frequently vaginal lacerations occur, although it is believed that they are relatively rare. In the majority of cases the vaginal lacerations occur during sexual acts consisting of penis, fist or object penetration of the vagina, particularly following a period of sexual inactivity,[23] and they have been described following both consensual and nonconsensual sexual acts. However, they have also been documented following vaginal instrumentation during the process of a medical assessment and following the use of plastic tampon inserters.[24] Lacerations have also been described following falls and a sudden increase of intraabdominal pressure, such as lifting a heavy object.[21]

Some females have obvious risk factors for vaginal lacerations (e.g. previous gynaecological surgery, congenital genital abnormalities, atrophic genital tissues, postmenopause, pregnancy and the puerperium) but the majority do not. Many theories have been postulated for why healthy females sustain vaginal lacerations during sexual intercourse. These include penile penetration of an unstimulated vagina[20] and genital disproportion, which is presumed to relate particularly to prepubertal and postmenopausal females.[25] However, the precise mechanism remains elusive.

It is not possible, from the cases reported in the literature, to determine how many times the penis entered the vagina before the reported vaginal laceration occurred, nor is it possible to determine the depth of penetration. It is also not possible to determine why some females sustained only single lacerations whereas others sustained multiple lacerations.

Injuries to the vagina have been noted during the examinations of complainants of sexual assault. These include tears, bruises, abrasions and redness, although the latter is a nonspecific finding with a number of causes.

If the vaginal laceration may have been caused by an object that has the potential to fragment or splinter, e.g. glass or wood, the wound should be inspected carefully for foreign bodies[26] and consideration given to undertaking a radiological assessment of the pelvis and vagina.[27] Any retrieved foreign bodies should be appropriately packaged and submitted for forensic analysis.

Cervix

Fraser et al.[19] noted petechiae on the forniceal surface of the cervix in the women examined within 24 hours of the vaginal intercourse.

Bruises and 'lacerations' of the cervix have been described following nonconsensual sexual acts.[3,28,29] The cervix can also be damaged by medical intervention. Confluent bruises and lacerations have not been described following consensual sexual acts.

Perianal area, anal canal and rectum

A significant proportion of complainants of sexual assault will have been subjected to penetration of the anus by an object, digit or penis. Therefore, the forensic practitioner must be familiar with the normal appearance of the perianal skin, the anal canal and the rectum.

Although frequently misused, the term anus simply refers to the external opening of the anal canal. The anus is surrounded by the perianal skin, which includes the folds of skin that radiate out from the anal 'margin' or 'verge'; these terms merely describe the skin adjacent to the anus at a given moment in time. When the anal sphincters are in the resting position, the perianal skin adjacent to the anal margin may appear pinker and shinier that the surrounding skin; this is particularly noticeable in young adults. The perianal skin is usually flesh coloured but it may be darker than the skin of the buttocks.

The perianal skin lies immediately over the anal sphincters that encircle the anal canal. When the buttocks are first separated, the external anal sphincter may be in its resting position whereby it encircles the lower end of the internal anal sphincter; if the perianal skin is palpated in this position it may be possible to identify both sphincters. However, the usual response to palpation (and even sometimes to the separation of the buttocks or inspection) is the voluntary or involuntary contraction of the external anal sphincter, which causes it to close like a purse string over the distal end of the internal sphincter so that some of the perianal skin recedes into the anal canal.

The anatomical anal canal extends from the 'anus' to the 'dentate line' (also referred to as the pectinate line). However, as discussed above, the anus and anal margins are not fixed points and sometimes the transition from the perianal skin to the lining of the anal canal is not clearly demarcated. The anal canal is lined by nonkeratinised squamous epithelium, which appears shiny and pink or red in the living. The 'dentate line' refers to an apparent 'line' formed either by the bases of the anal columns or, when these are not apparent, by the lowest visible anal sinuses.[30] In the living, these can be difficult to identify without magnification. The anatomical anal canal in females aged 18 years is short, measuring 1.0–3.2 cm.[31] There is no literature documenting the precise length of the anal canal in persons under the age of 18 years.

At the superior end of the anal canal is the anal transitional zone, which can appear purple in colour. Those inexperienced in proctoscopy could mistake this area for circumferential bruising. Superior to the anal transitional zone is the rectum, which is 8–15 cm long. The rectum is lined by typical intestinal mucosa and appears dark red in the living.[31] Both the perianal skin and the anal canal are sensitive to touch, pain, heat and cold.[30] The rectum has only poorly defined dull sensation.[30]

Following allegations of nonconsensual anal penetration, the most frequently detected injuries are anal fissures, tears and lacerations.[3,32] Use of different terminology hampers the interpretation of the injuries. McCann and Voris[33] have suggested that laceration of perianal skin should be described in terms analogous to those used to describe perineal tears following childbirth (Table 8.2).[34]

Table 8.2. Classification of laceration to perianal skin[33]

Degree of laceration	Description
First	Superficial laceration of the perianal skin or mucosa of the anal canal that may or may not be perpendicular to the anal verge. The underlying musculature may be exposed but there is no apparent damage to it
Second	Laceration of the perianal skin or mucosa of the anal canal which involves the underlying musculature
Third	Laceration of the perianal skin or mucosa of the anal canal which extends through the musculature into the anal canal or rectum

A fresh laceration may be bleeding or oozing, will have sharply demarcated edges and will not show any signs of healing such as reddening of the edges, induration, oedema and slough in the base of the wound. Although a forensic practitioner may be tempted to age precisely a laceration in an attempt to relate it dogmatically to a specific incident, this would be unwise, owing to the lack of information regarding the healing process in this area.

Whether an injury heals by primary or secondary intention depends upon a number of factors, including the width and depth of the breach in the epithelium and whether the trauma is acute or chronic. This distinction is somewhat arbitrary, as both processes involve both regeneration and repair, the latter resulting in scar tissue. However, when minor wounds heal, the scar tissue may not be identifiable externally[35] but it would be apparent if the area were biopsied and viewed microscopically.

In addition to lacerations, bruises, abrasions, oedema and erythema have all been noted on the perianal skin, epithelium of the anal canal and rectum of complainants of sexual assault.[3,18]

If there is little information regarding the genital injuries associated with consensual penovaginal penetration there is even less information regarding the perianal and anal canal and rectal injuries sustained during consensual penoanal penetration. This may be because it is unusual for injuries to occur or that the injuries are minor and, as such, are either not noticed by the complainant or not presented to a healthcare professional. There is one study that specifically attempted to address the medical complications experienced by 129 women who gave a history of anal intercourse.[36] This study found that only one woman described anal complications, namely proctitis and an anal fissure, but in fact both of these signs related to a gonococcal infection. However, as the study was limited to the medical history, it is not possible to rule out the presence of minor asymptomatic conditions or injuries in this study population.

Sohn and Robilotti[37] identified 18 (6.9%) men with anal fissures among 260 male homosexuals. However, first-degree anal lacerations (which, if perpendicular to the perianal margin, are also called fissures) have numerous nonsexual causes including constipation, skin disease and inflammatory bowel disease. On the basis of the present literature, in the absence of other abnormalities, it is not possible to differentiate between nonsexual and sexual causes of fissures.

There are numerous case reports describing perforating or nonperforating lacerations of the rectum following sexual acts.[38,39] However, many of these relate to object or fist penetration rather than penile penetration.[38,39] On occasion, the injury may be fatal.[38,39] Most case reports do not specify whether the sexual acts were consensual or not. Slaughter et al.[3] described five rectal lacerations among eight women who underwent proctoscopy following 'anal contact' during a sexual assault; the precise sexual act (i.e. penis, object etc.) is not described. There is also a case report describing a female who presented with perineal bruising, multiple superficial skin tears, an infected perineal wound and defects of both sphincters 48 hours after nonconsensual penoanal penetration with or without object penetration.[40]

The dilemmas

Determining consent for sexual acts

Clearly, it would be of immense value to the court if the nature and pattern of any genital injuries could differentiate between consensual and nonconsensual sexual acts. Slaughter et al.[3] conducted a study to see if this was possible. They compared the sites and numbers of the genital and anal injuries noted during the examination of 311 female subjects who made 'valid' complaints of sexual assault and with those noted during the examination of 75 women who were seen within 24 hours of 'consensual sexual intercourse'. The authors commented that "although coital injury seems to be associated with insertion of the penis its prevalence is significantly associated with a history of nonconsensual sexual intercourse". However, there are two problems with this study. Firstly, the complaint was classified as 'valid' if the police investigation corroborated the complainant's history and the complainant did not retract the allegation. Clearly, it is possible that some of the complainants of nonconsensual acts had, in fact, voluntarily engaged in the sexual acts. Secondly, 48 women out of the total of 75 in the 'consensual' group had been "evaluated initially as victims, but later changed their story to consensual sexual intercourse". If any of this group had continued to give a dishonest story and had not actually had recent sexual intercourse, this could have produced a biased result. Indeed, the authors conceded that "further investigation is needed to determine whether there is a finding or group of findings that can distinguish nonconsensual from consensual activity". Therefore, on the basis of the available literature, it is not possible to determine from the genital and anal injuries whether the sexual acts were consensual or nonconsensual.

Colposcopy and photodocumentation

A colposcope provides a convenient source of magnification (5x–30x) and illumination for the assessment of the external and, where relevant, the internal genital or anal areas of complainants of sexual assault. There are two main types available in the UK. The first is a binocular microscope that the operator uses to view the relevant areas directly. The second is a video colposcope that relays the image to a monitor. With the appropriate attachments, both systems allow the practitioner to obtain a truly contemporaneous, permanent, still or video record of the genital or anal findings. Use of a video recording system documents the entire genital examination and will show any dynamic changes. There are other types of equipment for recording the genital findings, such as conventional cameras and videos, but these do not have all the advantages of the colposcope and may not be acceptable to the complainant.

Advantages to the complainant

- The colposcope provides magnification and a cool light source to enable a rapid assessment of the genital and anal areas at a distance of around 30 cm (i.e. focal length of the system being used) from the area being inspected. In the author's experience, complainants find this more comfortable than being inspected by a hand-held lens that necessitates a much closer proximity between the practitioner and the complainant.

- Colposcopy significantly improves the detection of genital trauma in women aged 15 years and older compared with gross visualisation alone.[19,41]

- Photodocumentation may enable the practitioner to obtain a second opinion on the medical findings without the complainant being subjected to a further examination. This is particularly pertinent to young people who are often reluctant to be examined in the first instance.

- Many practitioners advocate the use of mirrors in children and young people to help them relax and become an active participant in the examination.[42] The colposcope with a monitor is an extension of this. Some children and young people choose to watch the monitor throughout the assessment. When appropriate, the monitor, instantaneous still images and video records can be used to demonstrate the medical findings to the complainant and carer. Forensic practitioners report that some young people appear to appreciate the opportunity to have fears of genital disfigurement allayed by the use of this equipment.

- Photodocumentation enables the practitioner's work to be audited and peer reviewed. This is essential, given the implications of an inaccurate diagnosis.

- If the case proceeds to court, photodocumentation enables the medical evidence to be reviewed by medical experts for the defendant.

- Photodocumentation provides material for teaching, debate, publication and research.

Disadvantages

- Colposcopes and attachments are expensive.
- Practitioners must acquire the necessary knowledge and skill to enable adept use of the equipment and the interpretation of the findings.
- Currently, there are only a few studies regarding the colposcopic findings following consensual sexual acts.
- Regular use of a conventional video recording system rapidly creates storage problems.

Consent

It is essential that colposcopy and photodocumentation are only used with the express consent of the complainant or carer. In obtaining consent, the practitioner must explain how any photodocumentation will be used and stored and to whom it could be disclosed. Complainants can be given the option to have a routine macroscopic assessment, a colposcopic assessment without photodocumentation or colposcopy with photodocumentation. As with all aspects of the assessment, the complainant retains her right to withdraw consent at any time during the consultation (see Chapter 4).

Use of stains

Many American forensic texts and protocols advocate the use of stains as an adjunct to the genital assessment of a complainant of sexual assault. The stain most frequently referred to is toluidine blue, which is a nuclear stain that was originally used in the 1960s to outline putative cervical and vulval neoplasia.[43,44] However, Lugol's solution has also been used in this context.[10] Like the colposcope, these stains have the potential to identify lacerations of the keratinised squamous epithelium that were not apparent on gross visualisation.[7,8] Toluidine blue may also show diffuse uptake within inflamed tissues and at excoriated and eroded sites.[8]

In the forensic context, vulval swabs must be taken before the stain is applied. Toluidine blue (1%) is then painted on the posterior fourchette, using a swab, prior to using a speculum. The residual stain is removed with lubricating jelly and gauze a few seconds after application.[8]

The advantage of using toluidine blue stain, in terms of enhancement of lacerations, must be balanced against the disadvantages:

- Application of the stain may cause localised discomfort.
- The stain will persist for some time, potentially causing embarrassment and acting as a stigma.
- Toluidine blue-positive posterior fourchette lacerations have been identified following consensual and nonconsensual penile penetration.[8,45]
- There is insufficient information regarding nonsexual causes for these superficial lacerations to attribute them just to sexual acts.

Conclusion

When relevant, complainants of sexual assaults should be offered a comprehensive assessment of the genital and anal areas, during which all injuries, potentially significant scars and medical conditions are noted and the necessary forensic samples obtained. Colposcopy may be a useful adjunct to the genital and anal assessment, in terms of identifying and recording fresh and old injuries and abnormalities. Toluidine blue and other stains may be useful to enhance injuries for photodocumentation. Further research is needed comparing the genital, anal and rectal injuries noted among complainants of sexual assault with those noted among the general sexually active population.

References

1. Ferrell J. Foley catheter balloon technique for visualising the hymen in female adolescent sexual abuse victims. *J Emerg Nurs* 1995;21:585–6.
2. Heger A, Emans S, Muram D. *Practice Guidelines in Evaluation of the Sexually Abused Child.* Oxford: Oxford University Press; 2000. Appendix F. p. 304.
3. Anatomy of the vulva and classification of disease. In: Leibowitch M, Staughton R, Neill S, Barton S, Marwood R. *An Atlas of Vulval Disease.* London: Martin Dunitz; 1997. p. 1–6.
4. Muram D. Anatomic and physiological changes. In: Heger A, Emans SJ, Muram D. *Evaluation of the Sexually Abused Child.* Oxford: Oxford University Press; 2000. p. 105–9.
5. Slaughter L, Brown, C, Crowley S, Peck R. Patterns of genital injury in female sexual assault victims. *Am J Obstet Gynecol* 1997;176:609–16.
6. Norvell M, Benrubi G, Thompson R. Investigation of microtrauma after sexual intercourse. *J Reprod Med* 1984;29:269–71.
7. McCauley J, Gorman R, Guzinski G. Toluidine blue in the detection of perineal lacerations in pediatric and adolescent sexual abuse victims. *Pediatrics* 1986;78:1039–43.
8. Lauber A, Souma M. Use of toluidine blue for documentation of traumatic intercourse. *Obstet Gynecol* 1982;60:644–5.
9. Biggs M, Stermac L, Divinsky M. Genital injuries following sexual assault of women with and without prior sexual intercourse experience. *Can Med Assoc J* 1998;159:33–7.
10. Bowyer L, Dalton M. Female victims of rape and their genital injuries. *Br J Obstet Gynaecol* 1997;104:617–20.
11. Examination of the vulva. In: Leibowitch M, Staughton R, Neill S, Barton S, Marwood R. *An Atlas of Vulval Disease.* London: Martin Dunitz; 1997. p. 7–12.
12. Kellog N, Parra J. Linea vestibularis: follow-up of a normal genital structure. *Pediatrics* 1993;92:453–6.
13. Jenny C, Kunhs M, Fukiko A. Presence of hymens in newborn female infants. *Pediatrics* 1987;80:399–400.
14. Royal College of Physicians of London. *Physical Signs of Sexual Abuse in Children.* London;1997.
15. Berenson A, Chacko M, Wiemann C, Mishaw C, Friedrich W, Grady J. A case–control study of anatomical changes resulting from sexual abuse. *Am J Obstet Gynecol* 2000:182:820–34.
16. Underhill R, Dewhurst J. The doctor cannot always tell: medical examination of the 'intact' hymen. *Lancet* 1978;i(8060):375–6.
17. Emans S, Woods E, Allred E, Grace, E. Hymenal findings in adolescent women: impact of tampon use and consensual sexual activity. *J Pediatr* 1994;125:153–60.
18. Adams J, Girardin B, Faugno D. Adolescent sexual assault: documentation of acute injuries using photo-colposcopy. *J Paediatr Adolesc Gynecol* 2001;14:175–180.
19. Fraser I, Lahteenmaki P, Elomaa K, Lacarra M, Mishell D, Alvarez F, *et al.* Variations

on vaginal epithelial surface appearance determined by colposcopic inspection of healthy, sexually active women. *Hum Reprod* 1999;14:1974–8.

20. Fish S. Vaginal injury due to coitus. *Am J Obstet Gynecol* 1956;72:544–8.

21. Metsala P, Nieminen U. Traumatic lesions of the vagina. *Acta Obstet Gynecol Scand* 1968;47:482–9.

22. Hoffman R, Ganti S. Vaginal laceration and perforation resulting from first coitus. *Pediatric Emergency Care* 2001;17(2):113–114.

23. Dia B, Diouf A, Bambara M, Bah MD, Diadhiou F. Les blessures vaginales au cours du coït: une série de 98 cas. *Contracept Fertil Sex* 1995;23:420–2.

24. Gray M, Norton P, Treadwell K. Tampon-induced injuries. Obstet Gynecol 1981;58:667–8.

25. Ahnaimugan S, Asuen M. Coital laceration of the vagina. *Aust N Z J Obstet Gynaecol* 1980;20:180–1.

26. Wilson F, Swartz D. Coital injuries of the vagina. *Obstet Gynecol* 1972;39:182–4.

27. Hakanson E. Trauma to the female genitalia. *Lancet* 1966;86:2286–91.

28. Burgess A, Holmstrom L. The rape victim in the emergency ward. *Am J Nurs* 1973;73:1741–5.

29. Slaughter L, Brown C. Cervical findings in rape victims. *Am J Obstet Gynecol* 1991;164:528–9.

30. Fenger C. Anal canal. In: Sternberg S, editor. *Histology for Pathologists*. 2nd ed. Philadelphia: Lippincott-Raven; 1997. p. 551–71.

31. Nivatovongs S, Stern H, Fryd D. The length of the anal canal. *Dis Colon Rectum* 1981;24:600–11.

32. Manser T. Findings in medical examinations of victims and offenders in cases of serious sexual offences – a survey. *Police Surgeon* 1991;38:4–27.

33. McCann J, Voris J. Perianal injuries resulting from sexual abuse: a longitudinal study. *Pediatrics* 1993;91:390–7.

34. Llewellyn-Jones D. *Fundamentals of Obstetrics and Gynaecology*. 3rd ed. London: Faber & Faber; 1982.

35. Amenta P, Martinez A, Trelstad R. Repair and regeneration. In: Damjanov I, Linder J, editors. *Anderson's Pathology*. 10th ed. St. Louis: Mosby; 1990.

36. Bolling D. Prevalence, goals and complications of heterosexual anal intercourse in a gynecologic population. *J Reprod Med* 1977;19:121–4.

37. Sohn N, Robilotti JG. The gay bowel syndrome. *Am J Gastrolenterol* 1977;67:478–84.

38. Crass R, Tranbaugh R, Kudsk K, Trunkey D. Colorectal foreign bodies and perforation. *Am J Surg* 1981;142:85–8.

39. Barone J, Yee J, Nealon T. Management of foreign bodies and trauma of the rectum. *Surg, Gynecol Obstet* 1983;56:453–7.

40. Engel A, Kamm M, Bartram C. Unwanted anal penetration as a physical cause of faecal incontinence. *Eur J Gastroenterol Hepatol* 1995;7:65–7.

41. Lenahan L, Ernst A, Johnson B. Colposcopy in evaluation of the sexual assault victim. *Am J Emerg Med* 1998;16:183–4.

42. Emans S, Goldstein D. *Pediatric and Adolescent Gynecology*. 3rd ed. Boston: Little Brown; 1990.

43. Richart R. A clinical test for the *in vivo* delineation of dysplasia and carcinoma *in situ*. *Am J Obstet Gynecol* 1963;86:703–11.

44. Collins C, Hansen L, Theriot E. A clinical stain for use in selecting biopsy sites in patients with vulvar disease. *Obstet Gynaecol* 1966;28:159–63.

45. McCauley J, Guzinski G, Welch R, Gorman R, Osmers F. Toluidine blue in the corroboration of rape in the adult victim. *Am J Emerg Med* 1987;5:105–8.

Chapter 9
Post-examination issues
Jan Welch

Introduction

Forensic examination following sexual assault is essential if evidence is to be collected for use in the investigation of crime. There are, however, other considerations at the initial examination and subsequently, so that risks to physical health are minimised and psychological recovery facilitated.

Survivors of sexual assault may have other injuries requiring attention as well as being at risk of pregnancy and sexually transmitted infections. The psychological trauma of the violation is commonly compounded by concerns about immediate and future safety, especially if the assault took place at or near the victim's home. Complainants of sexual assault frequently need help not only from the police and forensic medical examiners but also from other statutory and voluntary providers of health and psychosocial care. Good links between all those involved will prevent the delays and inconsistencies that otherwise aggravate the disempowerment associated with the initial assault, and perhaps delay recovery.

First aid

General body trauma is more common than genital trauma in association with rape and sexual assault. In Riggs *et al.*'s series of 1076 cases,[1] 64% of all sexual assault victims had general body trauma, with the extremities most commonly injured, followed by the head and neck; 53% had evidence of genital trauma and 20% had no injuries documented.

Other physical injuries are rarely severe, although occasionally assessment of major trauma, such as head injury, or examination and suturing of genital injuries under anaesthesia is required. If the complainant is to be anaesthetised then samples for forensic examination and photographs should if possible be taken, with consent, at the same time.

Minor physical injuries are common and may require medical attention. Nineteen percent of the cases in Riggs' study[1] needed additional medical procedures or interventions, such as plain X-rays, computed tomography scans of the head and abdomen, urinalysis, haematocrit measurement or suturing. Ideally, facilities for dressing of minor injuries and tetanus prophylaxis etc. should be available at the site of the initial examination, rather than the complainant needing to attend an accident and emergency unit for additional treatment.

Emergency contraception

Emergency postcoital contraception should be considered for all women following rape. In the USA, the rape-related pregnancy rate has been estimated at 5.0% per rape among those of reproductive age.[2] In one sample, of 34 cases of rape-related pregnancy, 47% had received no medical attention related to the rape and 32% did not discover they were pregnant until the second trimester; the majority were adolescents.

The most suitable method of emergency contraception will depend upon the patient profile, the time since the assault and the timing of any unprotected intercourse. The sooner that emergency contraception is started, the greater the efficacy.[3] A single dose (two tablets) of levonorgestrel 1.5 mg, started as soon as possible within 72 hours, is an effective and well-tolerated regimen, although the woman should be advised that no contraceptive method is 100% reliable. Evidence suggests that it is of value up to 120 hours after unprotected intercourse.[3]

Insertion of a copper-containing intrauterine contraceptive device (IUCD) is highly effective in preventing pregnancy and should be considered for women presenting after 72 hours but within five days (120 hours) after their most likely expected date of ovulation, based upon their previous shortest cycle length. Antibiotic prophylaxis to cover gonorrhoea and *Chlamydia trachomatis* should be considered,[4] especially following high-risk assaults such as those involving multiple assailants. An emergency IUCD is significantly more effective in preventing pregnancy than hormonal postcoital contraception and so, occasionally, this may be the method of choice for someone presenting within 72 hours since the rape, especially after mid-cycle rape. As IUCDs can often be inserted some time after the actual assault and the woman may change her mind about using this method, it may be appropriate to prescribe hormonal emergency contraception while waiting for an IUCD to be fitted.

Sexually transmitted infections

Risk

Rape is potentially a major risk for transmission of sexually transmitted infection (STI) and addressing these risks can allay most common concerns expressed by victims of sexual assault.[5] It is important to consider each person individually, as there may be substantial differences in their risks and concerns; for example, related to whether the assailant was a previous partner or a stranger. Although it is often impossible to determine whether the infection was pre-existing or acquired from the assault, STIs that are evident within 72 hours of the assault probably antedate it.[6] Studies of STIs in women who have been raped have shown rates of 3.9–56.0%, with the most common infections reported being those most commonly seen in the local community, including gonorrhoea, trichomoniasis and *C. trachomatis*.[7] STIs are often multiple, and the finding of one infection should prompt the search for more. A significant proportion of these infections are not identified on initial investigation but only diagnosed at follow-up.[8,9]

As with all laboratory tests, those for STIs carry a small chance of being incorrect. Errors may occur at any stage, from collection and labelling of the sample, to analysis and reporting. Investigations are neither 100% sensitive nor 100% specific, meaning that they may occasionally fail to pick up an infection which is present (false negative) or give a positive result when no infection is present (false positive). It is therefore good practice to confirm results by repeating tests that have major implications for the client (for example, a positive HIV test) or when the initial result seems improbable.

CASE 1

A nine-year-old girl had an accident on her bicycle, which resulted in minor genital trauma. A few days later some discharge was noticed on her underwear and she was taken to see her GP. Swabs were taken, including one for chlamydia. A positive result for chlamydia was telephoned to the surgery; social services were alerted and the child was taken into care pending further assessment. Detailed investigation found no evidence of abuse and a repeat test for chlamydia was negative.

STIs and evidence

Good notes and documentation are essential, even if the complainant does not plan to involve the police, as sometimes this will change and a statement may be requested some time later. In addition, forms may need to be completed to support criminal injuries compensation and this is much harder if good contemporaneous notes are not available. The use of a pro forma for those presenting following rape, for example to a sexual health service, is invaluable, both in ensuring that all relevant information is documented and to influence care provision by inexperienced staff.

In a sexually active complainant of rape, the diagnosis of an STI is seldom useful in court, as it can be used by the defence to denigrate her character. In such circumstances it is important, therefore, to separate the forensic notes from those used in the management of STIs and to ensure that different doctors are involved, to avoid conflict of interest in court.

Laboratory diagnosis and chain of evidence

The diagnosis of an STI may be relevant evidence in the sexually inexperienced and at the extremes of age. If the results of investigations are likely to be used medico-legally, attention should be paid to the types of tests used and the management of the sample. If possible, this process should be discussed in advance with local laboratories and a policy drawn up to cover arrangements for medico-legal samples. Tests used should ideally be well validated for medico-legal use and capable of confirmation, such as culture for gonorrhoea and chlamydia. Fewer laboratories now provide chlamydia culture, however, as newer more sensitive investigations such as nucleic acid amplification tests (NAATs) are adopted. Although medico-legal experience with NAATs is currently limited, such tests are increasingly well validated for routine practice and carrying out a confirmatory test from the original sample may be feasible.

The sample should be accompanied to the laboratory by a form documenting the chain of evidence: details of the sample, when and where it was taken, by whom and from whom, and a record of everyone handling the sample in its journey. This process should continue in the laboratory, where laboratory investigations should be supervised by senior staff who can arrange for additional confirmatory and other tests, as well as being well prepared to give evidence should this prove necessary. In the case of gonorrhoea, for example, it is essential that isolates are saved in duplicate locally, ideally at −70°C, or sent promptly to the reference laboratory to ensure adequate storage in addition to typing. Typing is invaluable in the unusual circumstance of gonorrhoea also being isolated from the alleged assailant, as it enables comparison between the two isolates.

Diagnosis and management

Potential visits and investigations are summarised in Box 9.1. Many women, however, do not wish to attend repeatedly and it is important to respect this in planning follow-up.

Before carrying out any genital examination it is important to consider the woman's comfort and feelings. A clear explanation should be given about what the examination entails and why it is necessary. If at all possible a female doctor should be offered; a male doctor should be supported by a female chaperone. Privacy is crucial; ideally there will be curtains round the examination couch to ensure this even if the examination room door is opened. Insertion of a cold speculum is uncomfortable for the woman and may increase her anxiety; this can be avoided if the speculum is warmed with tap water. See also Chapter 8.

Box 9.1

Medical care following rape

This is an idealised schedule, which should be adapted as necessary to meet the needs and wishes of the complainant.

Initial presentation (e.g. for forensic examination)

■ Psychosocial support
■ Consider post-coital contraception
■ Consider post-exposure prophylaxis for HIV (PEP) and hepatitis B
■ Discuss follow-up arrangements
■ Consider prophylactic antibiotics if declines follow-up

First health check (3–10+ days after assault)

■ Post-coital contraception/post-exposure prophylaxis follow-up
■ Offer genital screen for infection (samples for gonorrhoea, chlamydia, trichomoniasis) plus pelvic examination if indicated
■ Offer prophylactic antibiotics if declines above or further examinations
■ Consider starting hepatitis B vaccination
■ Baseline syphilis serology; HIV serology if taking post-exposure prophylaxis
■ Serum save (usually stored in virology, can be tested in parallel with later samples for HIV and hepatitis B and C)
■ First meeting with counsellor or health adviser; offer further counselling

Second health check (2 weeks later)

■ Post-coital contraception/post-exposure prophylaxis follow-up
■ Give results of previous tests
■ Offer repeat genital screen for infection
■ Discuss subsequent follow up

Third health check (3 months after assault)

■ Pre-test discussion for HIV, syphilis; offer tests
■ Psychosocial support/offer further counselling

Final health check (6 months after assault)

■ Pre-test discussion for hepatitis B and C, offer tests
■ Offer additional HIV test if high-risk incident; offer further counselling

Initial presentation

To avoid conflict of interest, at the time of forensic examination it is usually not appropriate to carry out diagnostic tests for STIs. It is, however, important to consider risk assessment and prophylaxis for HIV and hepatitis B if indicated (see sections below).

If a woman is unable, unwilling or unlikely to return for follow-up, the use of empirical prophylactic antibiotics should be considered, depending upon the wishes of the woman and the risks of the assault. The aim is to prevent gonorrhoea and chlamydial infection and their serious sequelae, such as pelvic inflammatory disease. There is little evidence of the efficacy of prophylaxis but national guidelines[4] recommend the use of: ciprofloxacin 500 mg plus azithromycin 1 g immediately; or ciprofloxacin 500 mg immediately plus doxycycline 100 mg twice a day for seven days or, if pregnant or breastfeeding: amoxicillin 3 g immediately plus probenecid 1 g immediately plus erythromycin 500 mg twice a day for 14 days.

First health check

If the police have been investigating a case of rape, the woman concerned is likely to have not only undergone a forensic examination but may also have spent many hours giving a detailed statement. Assessment for STIs is therefore best deferred until a week or so after the assault. At follow-up, avoidance of waiting, privacy and a supportive environment are crucial in minimising additional trauma.

Many women are happy to have a full genital examination and samples taken for infections, providing that this is done sensitively. Others may feel that the examination is an additional violation, in which case the use of prophylactic antibiotics should be considered, as above. As even one full set of investigations will miss up to12–15% of STIs, prophylactic antibiotics should also be considered for women unwilling to return for a further set of tests, especially following high-risk incidents such as group rape.

At this visit, samples should be taken for gonorrhoea (ideally swabs for culture from cervix, urethra, rectum, and throat if fellatio occurred), chlamydia (method depends on local methods available; ideally a cervical sample) and trichomoniasis (high vaginal sample). NAATs for chlamydia and gonorrhoea are becoming increasingly available and may be much more acceptable to the woman, since they can be carried out on a urine test or perineal swab. Baseline syphilis serology should also be taken and a sample stored in the laboratory for later testing, should the woman subsequently be found to have HIV or viral hepatitis, in order to assist in dating seroconversion.

Subsequent health checks

Subsequent health checks enable follow-up of earlier treatment, such as postcoital contraception, anti-bacterial and antiviral prophylaxis, as well as opportunities for further psychosocial support and referral, where necessary, and STI screening including serology after three to six months (Table 9.1).

Role of genitourinary medicine

Departments of genitourinary medicine or sexual health are generally well placed to offer both support to those who have been sexually assaulted and advice to those providing acute care and forensic examination. Most genitourinary medicine clinics can fast-track complainants of sexual assault, so that they can be seen promptly on the next day that the clinic is open. Genitourinary medicine services routinely offer advice about and screening for all likely infections and will provide free treatment for and assistance in the interpretation of any infections found. Their health advisers will generally be able to provide immediate and continuing psychosocial support, as well as information about other local sources of support and referral as necessary.

CASE 2

A fifteen-year-old girl was taken to her GP with abdominal pain. She had been withdrawn and moody for the previous few months, which her mother ascribed to her age. The GP took a careful history and elicited that the girl had been raped a few months before by four boys from the estate where she lived. She had been too frightened and ashamed to tell anyone before. She was referred to the local genitourinary medicine service, where she felt able to talk to a health adviser about what had happened and her feelings. She then felt able to have a genital and pelvic examination and swabs taken. Bimanual examination showed cervical excitation and bilateral adnexal tenderness and she was given antibiotics for pelvic inflammatory disease. Chlamydia was later identified. She received several sessions of support from the health adviser and later decided that she wished to talk to the police about what had happened.

Hepatitis B

Hepatitis B acquisition following rape has been described[10] but it is uncommon. National guidelines recommend that hepatitis B vaccine should be offered to all victims of sexual assault.[4] It is not known how long after the assault this may be effective but, as hepatitis B has a long incubation period, it may be of value up to three weeks later. It can be given as a 0-, 1- and 6-month regimen, with the final dose carried out at the same time as serologic testing, or as an accelerated course at 0, 1 and 2 months, with a booster at 12 months; or 0, 7 and 21 days, with a booster at 12 months.

If there is an especially high risk associated with the assault (for example, trauma with multiple assailants) or the assailant (for example, known to be an injecting drug user or from a high prevalence area such as the Far East or Africa) and rapid protection is required, an accelerated course of hepatitis B vaccine should be started as soon as possible after exposure and within 72 hours and consideration given to the use of hepatitis B hyperimmune globulin in addition.[11]

Healthcare workers and some other groups (injecting drug users, sex workers, some travellers) may have already been vaccinated against hepatitis B. If so, then a full vaccination history should be taken and immunity checked.

Psychosocial support

There is significant physical and mental health morbidity associated with sexual assault and survivors require appropriate care, information and continuing support (see Chapter 12).

At the time of the initial examination, a sensitive and supportive environment is essential but formal counselling is generally inappropriate, as most complainants are acutely traumatised from the initial assault, as well as being exhausted from lack of sleep and from necessary police interviews. Practical and emotional support from trusted members of her family, and friends, can be invaluable and women should be encouraged to seek such help, as well as involving their GPs as necessary. Information about local support and counselling agencies should be provided in writing, so that this is readily available should the woman wish to access support months or years later.

HIV post-exposure prophylaxis

Drugs to minimise the risk of acquiring HIV infection after rape are given in many countries where the prevalence of HIV is higher than in the UK. There is no direct evidence of efficacy, and the drugs are hard to take and expensive. Should they be offered?

The dilemma relates both to individual women and to healthcare services, as, at present in the UK, healthcare provision following rape is patchy and it may be extremely difficult to access drugs and expertise to provide immediate post-exposure prophylaxis for HIV, especially at night. If post-exposure prophylaxis is to be offered as part of a service, arrangements for this should be made in advance.

Risks of the assault

Concerns about HIV infection are common for those who have been raped. A reassuring discussion emphasising the smallness of the risk is therefore preferable to avoidance of the topic. The risk of acquiring HIV is minute in areas of low prevalence, such as the UK, but is likely to be higher if the rape took place in a high-prevalence area. It is important to consider each case individually.

A risk assessment can be carried out at the initial presentation following rape and, in our experience, this does not appear to add to distress provided

Table 9.1. Risk of seroconversion after a single exposure from an HIV positive source

Source	Risk of seroconversion (*n*)
Needle stick injury	1/270–300
Receptive vaginal intercourse	1/600–2000
Receptive anal intercourse	1/30–150

that it is carried out in a factual and reassuring manner. Risks can relate to the assault and the assailant. High-risk assaults are those involving factors including multiple assailants, genital trauma,[12] defloration or anal rape. Assailants at increased risk are those known or believed to have HIV, injecting drugs users, ex-prisoners, bisexual men and men from areas of the world where the prevalence of HIV is high (sub-Saharan Africa, the Caribbean, South and South-East Asia, parts of North and South America). Even if the assailant is unknown, in many cases (drug rape excepted) the complainant will be able to provide some information about him to assist in risk assessment.

The risk of seroconversion after a single exposure from an HIV positive source is shown in Table 9.1. The risk of the assault is increased by trauma and defloration, or if it involved multiple assailants.

Risks of the assailant

It is usually impossible to determine whether a rapist has HIV. The risk will depend upon the background prevalence of HIV and the presence of any additional risk factors. Estimated prevalence of HIV in the UK is shown in Table 9.2.

Example of individual risk of HIV

A woman has nonconsensual vaginal intercourse with an injecting drug user, without trauma. Her maximum risk would be:

$$\underset{\text{(chance of his having HIV)}}{1/30} \times \underset{\text{(risk of acquisition)}}{1/600} = 1/18\,000$$

This risk would be much higher, however, if the assault included the presence of trauma, anal rape and multiple assailants.

Table 9.2 Estimated prevalence of HIV in the UK

Population	Prevalence of HIV (*n*)
Overall	1/300–4000
Injecting drug users	1/30–500
Man from high-prevalence area, e.g. sub-Saharan Africa	1/30–60
Homosexual or bisexual man	1/50+

HIV prevention

There is evidence for the efficacy of post-exposure prophylaxis against HIV following occupational exposure[13] and in babies born to HIV-infected women, but not following sexual exposure or assault. Most of the evidence that does exist is based on the use of a single drug, zidovudine, but two or even three drugs are now routinely used to maximise efficacy, especially if resistant virus might be present. The drugs are started as soon as possible after exposure, ideally within an hour, and are continued for four weeks, at a cost of about £600.

In Wiebe *et al.*'s study,[14] in Canada, 258 people who presented to an emergency department following sexual assault were offered HIV prophylaxis. Of these, 71 accepted but only 29 continued with the drug treatment after receiving the initial five-day starter pack and only eight completed the full course and returned for follow-up.

Those at high risk of HIV infection were found to be more likely to accept prophylaxis and more likely to complete the treatment than those at lower risk. After this evaluation, the service changed its policy to offer HIV prophylaxis only to people thought to be at high risk of HIV infection.

Anti-retroviral drugs currently recommended in the UK for post-exposure prophylaxis[15] and commonly used for this purpose are: zidovudine 250 mg twice a day; plus lamivudine 150 mg twice a day (these two drugs can be given as a combined tablet; Combivir®, Glaxo SmithKline); plus nelfinavir 1250 mg twice a day (five tablets, taken with food).

Ideally, these drugs should be started within hours of the assault; significant benefit is much less likely if they are started after 72 hours. Antiemetic and anti-diarrhoeal medication should also be considered, as adverse effects include nausea, vomiting, headaches and gastrointestinal adverse effects such as diarrhoea. There may also be reduced efficacy of oral contraceptives. In addition, taking regular medication may perpetuate distress by serving as a reminder of the assault.

The medication is difficult to take and it is usual to give a 'starter pack' of drugs for three to five days, then review, as many people will choose not to continue on the medication. A physician with experience in the use of anti-retroviral drugs should monitor those who continue to take the treatment for the full four weeks. HIV testing following a pre-test discussion should be recommended at baseline and after six months.

When should HIV post-exposure prophylaxis be considered?

Given the above, it seems wise to carry out a risk assessment for HIV routinely, but to consider recommending post-exposure prophylaxis only following those incidents perceived to be carrying a high risk. These would include the presence of one or more of the following:

■ assailant known to have HIV
■ assailant in risk group
■ anal rape
■ trauma and bleeding
■ multiple assailants.

Prophylaxis is most likely to be effective if started within 72 hours.

References

1. Riggs N, Houry D, Long G, Markovchick V, Feldhaus KM. Analysis of 1076 cases of sexual assault. *Ann Emerg Med* 2000;35:358–62.
2. Holmes MM, Resnick HS, Kilpatrick DG, Best CL. Rape-related pregnancy: estimates and descriptive characteristics from a national sample of women. *Am J Obstet Gynecol* 1996;175:320–4.
3. Faculty of Family Planning and Reproductive Health Care, Royal College of Obstetricians and Gynaecologists. *FFPRHC Guidance: Emergency Contraception.* London: FFP; April 2003 (updated June 2003). [www.ffprhc.org.uk/clinical_effect/EC%20revised%20PDF%2019.06.03.pdf]. Accessed 1 September 2003.
4. Clinical Effectiveness Group (Association of Genitourinary Medicine and the Medical Society for the Study of Venereal Diseases). National Guidelines on the Management of Adult Victims of Sexual Assault. 2001. [www.agum.org.uk/ceg2002/sexassault0601.htm]. Accessed 1 September 2003.
5. Holmes M. Sexually transmitted infections in female rape victims. *AIDS Patient Care* 1999;13(12):703–8.
6. Girardin BW, Faugo DK, Seneski PC, Slaughter L, Whelan M. Findings that result from non-assault injury, infection, and other non assault variations. *Color Atlas of Sexual Assault.* St Louis: Mosby; 1997. p. 67–82.
7. Lamba H, Murphy SM. Sexual assault and sexually transmitted infections: an updated review. *Int J STD AIDS* 2000;11:487–91.
8. Estreich S, Forster GE, Robinson A. Sexually transmitted diseases in rape victims. *Genitourin Med* 1990;66:433–8.
9. Jenny C, Hooton TM, Bowers A, Copass MK, Krieger JN, Hillier SL, *et al.* Sexually transmitted diseases in victims of rape. *N Engl J Med* 1990;323:1141–2.
10. Crowe C, Forster GE, Dinsmore WW, Maw RD. A case of acute hepatitis B occurring four months after multiple rape. *Int J STD AIDS* 1996;7:133–4.
11. Brook MG. Sexual transmission and prevention of the hepatitis viruses A–E and G. *Sex Transm Infect* 1998;74:395–8.
12. Claydon E, Murphy S, Osborne EM, Kitchen V, Smith JR, Harris JR. Rape and HIV. *Int J STD AIDS* 1991;2:200–1. 1991.

13. Cardo DM, Culver DH, Cjesielski CA, Srivastova PU, Marcus R, Abiteboul D, *et al.* A case–control study of HIV seroconversion in health care workers after percutaneous exposure. *N Engl J Med* 1997;337:1485–90.

14. Wiebe ER, Comay SE, McGregor M, Ducceschi S. Offering HIV prophylaxis to people who have been sexually assaulted: 16 months experience in a sexual assault service. *CMAJ* 2000 162:641–5.

15. UK Health Departments. *HIV Post-exposure Prophylaxis: Guidance from the UK Chief Medical Officer's Expert Advisory Group on AIDS.* London: Department of Health; July 2000. [www.doh.gov.uk/eaga/pepgu20fin.pdf] Accessed 1 September 2003.

Chapter 10

The statement

Helen Cameron

Introduction

The guiding principles when providing a statement for police and the Crown Prosecution Service (CPS) is that the document should contain only forensic information together with any other information that is likely to affect the outcome of the case. Very little is known about the role of medical evidence in the legal resolution of sexual assault cases and Du Mont and Parnis question the value of uncritically collecting medical forensic evidence.[1] The preparation of a well-constructed statement with carefully considered interpretations and conclusions that may answer all of the potential questions in court might negate the need for a personal appearance in the witness box. Being called to court can be a frustrating, time-consuming experience with frequent delays and inevitable interference with day-to-day clinical practice.

Types of statement

The minimum requirement for a doctor's statement is in the form of a 'professional witness to the fact' document providing a factual account of the examination and a basic interpretation of the findings. It is the usual practice for an expert witness to be called to provide an opinion in a case where he or she has not been involved in the clinical examination. In the preparation of a statement by a relatively new forensic medical examiner, the advice of an experienced examiner might be sought.

Use of record of medical and forensic examination

Doctors undertaking forensic medical examination will usually have access to a document in which to record the details of the examination. This record should be completed contemporaneously. A list of the forensic specimens taken should also be kept. Since the Northumbria Police Record of Medical Examinations was first used in 1983, there have been many alterations to the style and content to accommodate changes in certain elements of the examination and forensic techniques. This form of record will assist the forensic medical examiner in the production of the statement.

Timing of statement preparation

It is a wise practice to complete a statement as soon as possible after the examination and to include an interpretation and opinion at the end of the statement, either using lay terminology where possible or, alternatively, providing a glossary of the medical terminology.

Aims of the statement
- Documentation of findings – normal or abnormal
- Causation of injuries
- Mechanisms leading to injury
- Degree of force required to produce the injury
- Other possible causes for findings
- Exclusion of unlikely causes
- Consistency of findings
- Opinion, using a sliding scale to describe the degree of certainty

Details of statement
- Core data:
- Qualifications, as a medical practitioner and any postgraduate awards
- Experience, such as current appointment and the nature of the job
- Previous relevant jobs or experience
- Special interests, indicating any other fields of experience
- Service on relevant local, regional or national committees
- Number of cases examined: this can be an optional field, especially for new forensic medical examiners.

That there has been an explanation of the role of the examining doctor:
- Have explained to the complainant the purpose of the examination
- Have obtained written consent for:
  - ☐ the forensic medical examination
  - ☐ any necessary photographs that may form part of the report and which may be revealed in subsequent court proceedings
- Have checked the medical needs of the complainant
- Have undertaken a physical examination
- Have collected samples that may be submitted for forensic testing
- It is usual to acknowledge that one's original notes can be made available for the assistance of any other doctor, be they instructed by the prosecution or the defence and that the statement has been prepared for use during any criminal trial.

Relevant medical, surgical, psychiatric history

Information collected solely in the context of providing medical care that is not germane to the case should not be included in the report. Continuing medical and surgical conditions requiring treatment should be mentioned, together with any disabilities. From an obstetric point of view, one should record the number and mode of deliveries that the woman has experienced. Problems with relevance of this information are discussed below.

Incident

This is usually in the form of an account of events from the complainant and the police officer. One should bear in mind that attempts to record all the specific details of the assault may hinder the prosecution if subtle historical contradictions are present. With regard to weapon use, the forensic medical examiner should document whether a weapon was used, as this may help to direct the investigator to look for specific injuries or potential areas of injury and allow substantiation of the complainant's allegation.[2] The presence of an injury is concrete evidence that something has indeed happened but the absence of injury must also make the forensic medical examiner consider, and include, a comment as to whether the complainant was threatened in any way.

Loss of evidence may be caused by a delay in presentation and so particular attention should be paid to the time interval since the incident.

Action taken by complainant affecting forensic evidence gathering and analysis

It is also important to consider the following factors both at the time of the examination and in preparation of the statement:

- details of the complainant's cleansing since event
- change of sanitary protection if menstruating
- eating and drinking
- teeth cleaning
- hair washing.

Details of examination

Judge the complainant's reaction to the examination; describe her demeanour, her mental state and attention (affect), her mood and whether she appears to be paying attention. With respect to her general appearance, her build, level of hygiene and state of nutrition might usefully be included.

The clothes that the complainant was wearing at the time of the incident should be listed if they are being seized by the forensic medical examiner to be submitted as the forensic medical examiner, rather than police, exhibits.

The presence of injuries should be carefully recorded and the injuries numbered on submitted diagrams; there should be a full description of the injuries (see below). If no injuries are found then there should be a comment to this effect.

Details of genital examination

Describe the complainant's reaction to examination, again describing demeanour during the procedure. Record whether or not there is evidence of trauma, bleeding or discharge or fluids seen at the various sites. Details of the instruments used, together with a standard description of the particular instrument and the role it plays in assessing the relevant genital area, should be included.

The standard instruments used are the vaginal speculum, proctoscope and colposcope, with or without video or camera attachment.

Glossary of anatomical terms used to describe genital sites

A glossary should be included in each case to assist not only the judiciary but also members of the jury at trial. Even the most obvious anatomical landmark, such as the anus, should be described in lay terms. It is often helpful to use colloquial terms such as the following descriptions:

■ vagina	front passage
■ anus	opening to the back passage
■ rectum	back passage
■ labia	lips to the vagina
■ fourchette or vestibule	entrance to the vagina
■ perineum	bridge of skin between the front passage
■ cervix	neck of the womb found inside the vagina
■ hymen	membrane that stretches across the opening to the vagina inside the vestibule or fourchette. Emphasise that the degree of completeness of the hymen varies between individuals.

Written description of injuries

When completing the statement the forensic medical examiner may experience difficulty with the nomenclature to describe wounds and may feel overwhelmed by the medico-legal significance of the lesions when challenged in the witness box, especially when asked to give an opinion as to the causation; see Chapter 11.

The description within the text should thus include whether or not all the potential types of wounds were present. It is also important to record everything that one expected to find but also that which was conspicuous by its absence. For bruises, the appearance in terms of size, colour, pattern, site and associated injuries should be documented. Similarly, the dimensions, pattern, site, active bleeding and associated injuries should be listed for abrasions, lacerations, incisions and stab wounds. One should record any evidence of healing of the injuries. Metric measurements should be used throughout.

Where the complainant has been severely injured, her medical needs must take priority over the need to achieve forensic samples. Where examination has taken place after suturing or surgery there should be a clear record of treatment received. If is not possible to gain access to an injury due to dressings etc., details of treatment should be obtained from the relevant clinicians (who should be warned that they too may be asked for a statement).

Clinical injury extent scoring

McGregor *et al.*[3] devised a 'clinical injury extent scoring' categorising injuries as none, mild, moderate or severe, based upon observed genital and extragenital injury. Criteria for clinical injury scoring were devised; for example, one of the criteria for a moderate injury score was 'injury or injuries expected to have some impact on function'. It was found to have good interobserver reliability and the results supported the hypothesis that there is an association between the laying of charges and the presence of documented moderate or severe injury. Thus, this study does provide evidence that the time spent on documenting the forensic part of the examination in the statement does influence the legal outcome of the case.

Use of standardised labelled diagrams

Use clock-face representation to describe the site of the injury. The diagrams should include the complainant's name, the date of examination and the doctor's signature.

Patterns of injuries

Some female survivors of sexual assault sustain more physical injuries than others and factors influencing the type of injury include the complainant's age and skin fragility. Genital trauma is more common in older women.[4,5] Where there are multiple bruises, it is essential to undertake a collective assessment of both the bruises and any other surrounding injury in an attempt to reconstruct events.[6] It is also important to recognise particular patterns of injury; for example, finger-tip bruising consisting of a row or a pair of circular or oval bruises, suggesting the blunt force of gripping associated with resistance in areas such as the upper arms, breasts and legs.

Samples submitted

A list of samples submitted for forensic examination should be included. This list may have been prepared by the accompanying police officer on the samples reference form, with the samples listed in the numerical order that they were seized and using a prefix of the forensic medical examiner's initials. A copy of this list is retained by the forensic medical examiner. Where a urine sample is submitted for drug analysis the time of voiding should be documented.

Post-examination arrangements

A comment should be made that the complainant has been offered appropriate medical advice, counselling and follow-up. Should the examination take place within a short time of the alleged incident, it may be appropriate to offer an appointment for re-examination in 48 hours, to allow any bruising to develop.

Interpretation of findings

As Rogers[7] has indicated, "the interpretation of the physical findings of complainants of sexual assault is one of the most difficult and controversial aspects of forensic medicine". The building of case experience is an important factor in developing expertise in forensic gynaecology but the legal profession, in particular, has an unrealistic expectation as to what conclusions can be reached following a forensic medical examination and the unwary forensic medical examiner may find themselves accused of bias. Thus, the most valuable examination in legal terms is one where the interpretation is undertaken by a forensic medical examiner with considerable experience in the examination of normal, diseased or traumatised genitalia who has a sound knowledge of the principles of injury interpretation.[8]

It is important to comment upon whether appearances of the genital area are normal or abnormal. In general, when considering bruises one should assess the site of the bruising and how this may affect the appearance of the bruise, and consider also the causation and the force of impact that might have caused the bruising. It is helpful to use a scale to describe one's degree of certainty about the likely cause of the particular injuries.

Suggested scale to describe the degree of certainty about causation

1   No suggestion that the injury is explained by, or relates to, any particular causation.

2   Mildly suggestive that the injury is explained by a particular causation.

3   Moderately suggestive that...

4   Strongly suggestive that...

5   Certainty that the injury has been caused by...

Conclusions

In preparing the conclusions, the overall causation and consistency needs to be addressed, so that the following aspects are covered:

- The presence of signs that **support** the allegation.
- Whether the signs are **consistent** with the allegation.
- The probable causation of the injuries.
- Whether or not consensual sexual activity could explain the findings.
- The effect of age and hormonal status on the genital tissues.
- The presence of any unusual injuries and the implication of such injuries.
- Reasons for absence of injury should be addressed in the conclusion; it is easy for counsel for the defence to highlight how unimpressive a case may look where there is absence of injury.
- Suggest realistic alternative causation, such as an accidental injury (e.g. streaky, linear bruising due to a watchstrap or piece of jewellery or an ovoid abrasion due to a fall against a similarly shaped object). The site of such injuries is important; for example, accidental bruising on the inner aspect of the thighs or knees is unlikely, a more likely cause being the blunt force of an assailant's knees or thumbs being applied to separate the legs.
- Inconsistencies: the possibility of a false allegation must be entertained when preparing the opinion. In interpreting any injury the doctor must consider whether it has any features suggestive of being self-inflicted. Clues that may assist in this assessment include the location of the wound (accessibility), the direction of linear, often parallel, scratches, the sparing of sensitive areas of the body.

The conclusion should end with a sentence indicating that the statement has been 'based on information given to me to date'. Also there should be some indication that modification of the conclusions may be necessary if further, relevant information becomes available.

Use of relevant references

The absence of genital injuries should not negate an allegation of sexual assault or rape but it does make it harder to prove to a jury. The presence of genital injury is thought to carry more weight in obtaining a successful conviction. With reported rates of visible genital injury that was apparent without special staining or magnification being between 16% and 27%, it is important that the examining doctor is able to quote published data to support the statement that the absence of genital injury does not imply consent by the complainant and that physical and genital injury are not an inevitable consequence of being raped.[9–11]

Final reminders

The police may provide the forensic medical examiner with printed statement forms but these are not mandatory. Those forensic medical examiners using word-processed statements, often with the aid of a template, should be aware that all statements in criminal cases must include a statutory declaration. In England and Wales, this should be along the following lines: "This statement, consisting of x pages, each signed be me, is true to the best of my knowledge and belief. I make it knowing that, if it is tendered in evidence, I shall be liable to prosecution if I have wilfully stated in it anything which I know to be false or do not believe to be true". The statutory declaration must be signed and dated.

Do ensure the statement has a professional appearance and final draft is checked carefully for errors. Each page should bear your signature at the foot of the page or at the end of the document if the page is not filled.

Dilemmas around the statement

Account of the events

How full an account of the events should be included in the doctor's record and statement? Forensic medical examiners should avoid playing detective; it is up to the police to obtain the detailed investigative history. Absolute impartiality is the rule in the preparation of the statement.

Recording the drug and alcohol consumption by the complainant may be interpreted by some as a potential character slur but is important to correlate the complainant's mental state and attention during the examination, together with the amount of voluntary alcohol or drug consumption. The use of drugs in 'date' or acquaintance rape is an increasingly common, with drugs such as flunitrazepam (Rohypnol®, Roche) being used to 'spike' drinks. Drugs impair the recollection of events surrounding the sexual assault, making identification and prosecution of the assailant even more difficult. A timed urine specimen should be considered where there are discrepancies between the declared amounts consumed and the complainant's behaviour.

Interpreting degree of force used from the complainant's account

The forensic medical examiner in the witness box is often challenged by Counsel for the Defence to interpret the degree of force used by the assailant. One particular question that the examiner should be prepared for is being asked whether or not the injuries could have resulted from consensual sexual intercourse. To avoid being embarrassed in court it is wise to address this issue in the context of the statement, indicating, if appropriate, that it is unlikely that such injuries would result from consensual intercourse since the force necessary to cause them would cause considerable pain and distress.

What is a 'relevant' medical and psychiatric history?

To avoid character slurs related to previous sexual history, one should avoid obstetric and gynaecological details such as a history of termination of pregnancy or sexually transmitted diseases and restrict the details to the number of children and mode of deliveries together with details of major gynaecological surgery.

Psychiatric problems requiring drug therapy or other interventions should be included as this may influence the complainant's account and behaviour during the examination. Likewise, learning and physical disabilities may contribute to difficulties with the forensic examination and need to be taken into consideration by the police, CPS and the court.

All medication, both prescribed and nonprescribed, taken in the days prior to the incident should be recorded.

Interpretation of the age of bruises

It is recognised that there are considerable difficulties in timing injuries by the colour of the bruises. The only reliable fact is that bruises with a yellow colour are more than 18 hours old and that the appearance of the other colours is less reliable.[12] Deep bruises can take 12–24 hours to appear.

Errors subsequently discovered in a signed submitted statement

Once the statement has been submitted, errors should be "corrected" with a supplementary signed statement. Even if the original statement has been returned, it is not possible to make charges using correction fluid. The minimum requirement then is to cross out the error in ink, make the alteration in handwriting, date and initial the correction.

Supporting new specialist forensic medical examiners

For a new forensic medical examiner, it is recommended that the statement is checked by an experienced examiner as soon as possible, as the full committal file may be served very rapidly; thus the police and the CPS need the supporting evidence and the forensic medical examiner's statement very quickly. A preface to the interpretation of the findings such as "I have discussed this case with Dr X prior to the preparation of this statement" may prove useful in these circumstances.

'Expert' witness statement

To improve the successful conviction rate and to provide a structure that is supportive to relatively inexperienced forensic medical examiners, the concept of a two-stage report in a single-contact case of sexual assault or rape has been proposed. The philosophy of such an approach is that the initial statement, made by the examining doctor who is a professional witness, is a factual account of the findings. For those cases likely to proceed to court, a second 'expert' statement might be commissioned. The initial forensic medical examiner might wish to end their initial conclusion with the following comment: "Should it appear likely that this case would proceed to court, a second, more detailed statement will be required." Either:

- I am prepared to provide that statement

  or

- An expert forensic medical examiner will prepare this statement.

As an expert, the doctor's legal position is one of an adviser to the prosecution on matters that are outside the experience of the general public. The expert should have access to the fullest possible picture in order to give the best advice and opinion. Accordingly, the expert should have sight of all relevant statements, a record of the defendant's interview, relevant medical records and the results of the scientific tests. Experts should prepare their statements based upon their analysis of the case and provide an opinion with the assistance of the first forensic medical examiner. It is recognised that an important factor in the development of expertise is the building of case experience and so, within the REACH organisation, we have established that an 'expert' forensic medical examiner is one who has examined 20 rape or sexual assault cases and has been actively involved as a forensic medical examiner for at least two years. In addition, the expert will have undertaken appropriate training and attended the REACH Scheme meetings and be an 'accredited' forensic medical examiner. The term 'accredited forensic medical examiner' implies that the examiner is willing and able to provide an expert statement. The ability to provide such a statement may depend upon the particular case in question. An accredited forensic medical examiner is under no obligation and the provision of an expert opinion is optional to those experienced enough to do so. Such a two-tier system may prove costly but with conviction rates running at about 10–15% internationally, this novel approach may assist the CPS in their assessment of the strength of a particular case.[13]

Role of documenting complainant's emotional state

Emotional state can be treated as a dichotomous variable: emotive if the complainant has been observed to be anxious, shaking or crying at the time of the examination and controlled if she was observed to be calm, detached or rational.[13] McGregor[13] found an even distribution of victims who presented as emotive (44.4%) versus controlled (47.6%), confirming that emotional responses to sexual assault are varied. She argues that there is no scientific basis for the examiner to document a victim's observed emotional response either as corroboration or noncorroboration of an allegation of sexual assault. Thus, by inference, it would appear that inclusion of the complainant's emotional state within the statement is questionable and its role warrants further evaluation.

Physician's role in interpretation of complainant's forensic test results

The chance of finding positive evidence from forensic testing is largely time-dependent, particularly regarding sperm and seminal products, which are weighted most heavily in rape investigations. The chances of recovering seminal evidence is less than 50%, with even lower chances after 24 hours.[14] It is important that all who work in the field of forensic gynaecology should understand that the absence of positive findings on forensic testing does not mean that no attack has taken place. Thus the physician and especially those acting as expert forensic medical examiners should be involved in the interpretation of a complainant's test results. In addition the forensic medical examiner's conclusions could contain an explanation of the likelihood of finding a positive result and allowing a greater emphasis to be placed upon the documented medical evidence.

Post-examination arrangements

Recommendation about re-examination, photography and odontology may also be included in the recommendation to the complainant. However, medical details such as the offer to screen for sexually transmitted diseases are best excluded from the report.

Conclusions

There is growing international concern about the low conviction rate for rape. The criminal justice systems in the USA and UK have introduced initiatives in an attempt to improve the response to rape cases. It is important to recognise that there is need for improvement in the forensic management of sexual assault cases including the interpretation of the examination findings. In preparing a statement, it is thus important to be aware of the possibility of subsequent legal involvement, paying particular attention to detail; this may prove beneficial if, and when, one is called to give evidence in court. The statement needs to be methodically prepared and the forensic medical examiner should avoid darting from one area to another. The opinion and conclusions must address the overall causation and consistency of the findings with the complainant's allegation but while being thorough the forensic medical examiner must remain impartial at all times and thus feel entirely comfortable in signing the statutory statement that accompanies each and every statement in England and Wales.

References

1. Du Mont J, Parnis D. Sexual assault and legal resolution: querying the medical collection of forensic evidence. *Med Law* 2000;19:779–92.
2. Gray-Eurom K, Seaberg DC, Wears RL. The prosecution of sexual assault cases: correlation with forensic evidence. *Ann Emerg Med* 2002;39:39–46.
3. McGregor MJ, Grace L, Marion SA, Wiebe E. Examination for sexual assault: is documentation of physical injury associated with the laying of charges? A retrospective cohort study. *CMAJ* 1999;160:1565–9.
4. Ramin SM, Satin AJ, Stone IC, Wendel GD. Sexual assault in postmenopausal women. *Obstet Gynaecol* 1992;80:860–4.
5. Cartwright PS, Moore RA. The elderly victim of rape. *S Afr Med J* 1989;82:988–9.
6. Vanezis P. Interpreting bruises at necropsy. *J Clin Pathol* 2001;54:348–55.
7. Rogers D. Physical aspects of alleged sexual assault. *Med Sci Law* 1996;36:117–22.
8. Lincoln C. Genital injury: is it significant? A review of the literature. *Med Sci Law* 2001;41:206-16.
9. Bowyer L, Dalton ME. Female victims of rape and genital findings. *Br J Obstet Gynaecol* 1997;104:617–20.
10. Cartwright PS, the Sexual Assault Study Group. Factors that correlate with injury sustained by survivors of sexual assault. *Obstet Gynaecol* 1987;70:44–6.
11. Cartwright PS, Moore RA, Anderson JR, Brown DH. Genital injury and implied consent to alleged rape. *J Reprod Med* 1986;31:1043–4.
12. Langlois NE, Gresham, GA. The ageing of bruises: a review and study of the colour changes with time. *Forensic Sci Int* 1991;50:227–38.
13. McGregor MJ, du Mont J, Myhr T. Sexual assault forensic examination: is evidence related to successful prosecution? *Ann Emerg Med* 2002;39:639–47.
14. Ferris LE, Sandercock J. The sensitivity of forensic tests for rape. *Med Law* 1998;17:333–49.

Chapter 11
The doctor in court

Raine Roberts

Introduction

Medical evidence in a rape case may be of crucial importance in determining whether a man receives a long prison sentence or whether guilty persons go unpunished. However, in many cases the doctor's evidence may only be a minor aspect of the case which may be purely an issue of consent.

It is important that the doctor is well trained in forensic medicine, aware of current medical literature and its limitations and able to give effective unbiased evidence.

The examination of rape complainants is very different from ordinary medical practice. While one must be a caring doctor and help the complainant appropriately, it is necessary to retain a degree of objectivity and not to feel that you must find evidence to support the complainant.

Usually a rape case will be heard in the Crown Court but, rarely, a complainant may bring a civil action, suing the alleged offender for damages.

Lord Justice Auld, in his review of the criminal justice system,[1] has recommended that medical evidence in criminal cases should follow guidelines similar to those well established in civil cases. These include a duty to assist the court on matters within the doctor's expertise. This duty overrides any obligation to the person from whom they have received instructions or by whom they are paid.

It is likely that the new criminal procedure rules recommended by Lord Justice Auld will require a declaration when any witness statement or report is prepared that it is for the assistance of the court.

It will increasingly be the case that, as in the civil courts, doctors involved in criminal cases will be expected to meet and reach a measure of agreement, identifying those issues on which they agree and those on which they do not agree and prepare a joint statement for use in evidence, indicating the measure of their agreement and a summary of the reasons for their disagreement.

Currently, in England and Wales but not in most other countries, any doctor can set him or herself up as an expert and give evidence in the type of case in which they have no direct relevant experience or no recent hands-on experience.

This will change in the near future when it is likely that doctors setting out to give expert evidence in the courts will have to be registered with the new Council for the Registration of Forensic Practitioners, which will set standards, assess performance and have an investigatory and disciplinary function.

What happens in a rape case?

Only in a proportion of cases where a complaint of rape has been made will a criminal prosecution be brought. The complainant may withdraw the allegation or the Crown Prosecution Service (CPS) may decide that there is insufficient evidence on which to proceed.

Under the terms of the Criminal Procedure and Investigations Act 1996, the officer investigating the case has a duty to establish what evidence should be put before the court and is required to see all the evidence in the case. There is still controversy within the medical profession as to whether the forensic medical examiner or police surgeon undertaking the rape examination is a member of the investigating team or is an independent third party. This point is relevant to the disclosure of contemporaneous notes. If the doctor is a member of the investigating team then the investigating officer must be provided with the contemporaneous notes at the same time as the witness statement. If the doctor is not a member of the investigating team then a note should be made in the witness statement that the notes will be provided to the CPS on request.

The contemporaneous notes are part of the evidence and must always be disclosed, preferably well before the date of the hearing. If the doctor does not disclose the notes but takes them to court on the day of the trial, this can lead to the case being adjourned with subsequent further stress on witnesses and further expenditure on public funds.

The CPS will then decide whether the case will go to court, using two criteria:

■ Is there a reasonable chance of a conviction?
■ Is the prosecution in the public interest?

The procedure may take many months and it is usually about six months before a case is heard in the Crown Court.

There is usually a preliminary hearing: the plea and directions hearing, to which the doctor is not called. Its purpose is to establish that the case is ready to be heard, the witnesses are available on the date to be set and to estimate a likely timescale for the hearing.

The defendant will enter his plea of guilty or not guilty. If he enters a plea of guilty he will be sentenced later at the Crown Court.

While a specific date is set for the hearing of a trial it may not be possible, for a variety of reasons, for the case to be heard on that date. A previous case may run over, key parties may be ill or have disappeared but eventually the case will start.

It is important in the interests of justice that the case should run in chronological order and while arrangements sometimes are made for doctors to give their evidence out of order, this is less satisfactory than if it is given in the proper sequence following the chronology of the events as they occurred.

The trial

1. The jury is sworn.
2. Prosecuting Counsel will outline the case (in Scotland this is not done and the case proceeds immediately to the hearing of the first witness). The Prosecution's opening speech may last from ten minutes to several hours, even days, usually outlining in considerable detail the evidence upon which the Crown will rely. Prosecuting Counsel will state to the jury that the Crown brings the case and it is for them to be sure, having heard all the evidence, whether the Defendant is guilty or not.
3. The complainant gives evidence.
4. The witnesses to whom the complaint was first made may give evidence next, or the doctor may be called to give an account of the medical examination.
5. The forensic scientist may be called with regard to DNA evidence.
6. Police officers will be called to describe their involvement in the case. The police officers will give an account of their tape-recorded interviews with the defendant. Usually this takes the form of a police officer reading out the questions they put to the defendant, with the Prosecution barrister playing the part of the defendant.
7. After the Prosecution case, the Defence will open its case. The Defence may or may not call witnesses. Since the law has been changed to allow juries to draw conclusions from a defendant not giving evidence, it is usually the case that the defendant will give his account of events.
8. If a Defence medical expert or a Defence forensic scientist is to be called, they will usually be called after the defendant.
9. There will then be closing speeches from the Prosecution and the Defence, followed by the Judge's summing-up, which will outline points of law and refer the jury to crucial areas in the evidence.
10. The jury will then retire and return if it reaches a unanimous verdict. If it is not able to reach a unanimous verdict after a period of time the Judge will recall the jury and tell them that he will accept a majority 10:2 verdict.

If the jury cannot reach a verdict then there may or may not be a retrial, depending upon the view of the CPS and perhaps the complainant.

A rape case is likely to last between three and four days. It is important for doctors to understand this and I would recommend that any doctor involved in the examination of rape complainants should try to attend the Crown Court and sit through a whole rape case, perhaps one where one of your colleagues is giving evidence. It can be illuminating to hear all the evidence in the case, which may look very different at that stage from the account given to the doctor on the night when the complainant was examined. It will also help in understanding the difficulties the court has in hearing the evidence at a time convenient to the doctor.

The prosecution doctor

The doctor who has examined the complainant is usually called by the Prosecution but, very rarely, the Defence may ask the doctor to attend.

The doctor is usually regarded as a professional witness and remunerated accordingly, but a doctor who has special expertise, training and qualifications, such as the Diploma in Medical Jurisprudence, may be recognised by the court as an expert and receive a higher fee.

How the case goes in court depends greatly upon how the examination has been conducted and recorded.

The examination and statement

Carry out a careful, thorough and appropriate examination, making careful and accurate notes. (see Chapters 6–8). It is necessary to establish with the complainant that the examination and its findings are for the purposes of a possible court case and that everything you have recorded may be seen by lawyers, other doctors and police officers (see Chapter 9).

Provide a statement, including an opinion as to the possible cause of the findings and considering other possibilities, or adding that you are prepared to consider such if they are put to you (see Chapter 10).

The week before the trial

Find out if there is a defence medical expert report. Insist on seeing it with sufficient time to prepare comments. Check that the case is still going on and is to be heard on the date set. Make sure that you know where the court is and how to get there.

The day before the trial

Read your notes and statement carefully, considering their weaknesses and strengths. Try to anticipate the questions that might be put in cross-examination and think through how you would deal with them. When you have done all this thoroughly, you may find that the really difficult questions are never put and you come out of the court feeling that you were not able to tell "the truth, the whole truth and nothing but the truth" because you were not asked the right questions. However, be assured that if you do not do your homework, the awkward questions will be put and unprepared or ill-thought-out answers may cause your evidence to lose much of its authority and impact.

The day of the trial

Allow yourself plenty of time to get to court; allow for traffic and parking. You may have a long wait, so take something to read. Remember to switch off your mobile telephone or pager: there is no point in making it more difficult for yourself in the court by annoying the judge. The classic advice to witnesses, as emphasised by the eminent forensic pathologist, Professor Bernard Knight, is: "to dress up, stand up, speak up, and shut up".[2]

Dress up

Giving evidence requires you to impress the court with your professionalism. There is no merit in turning up at court in a rugby shirt and trainers or in a sloppy floral frock, even if it is fashionable. A neat dark suit and a generally tidy appearance will make it easier for you to impress the court as a serious professional.

Stand up

The judge may invite you to sit down. I prefer to stand. I find it much easier to be able to listen to the questions put by the barristers and then talk to the jury or the judge, as appropriate. I feel much more in control of what I am saying if I am standing rather than sitting.

Speak up

You have to make sure that the whole court can hear what you are saying and I find this is best achieved by speaking across the court towards the back row of the jury. Your answers are directed to the judge and jury and not to the person who asked the question, the barrister, unlike in everyday life, where you answer the person speaking to you. Turn slightly to listen to the question and then turn back to answer it.

Shut up

This is the difficult one. Defence counsel may pause at the end of one of your answers and you may feel that you are expected to say more. This is a dangerous situation but do not be tempted to expand, exposing yourself to the danger of saying something that counsel can pick up on as being contradictory to something you said earlier.

There are often pauses during the giving of evidence while counsel and the witness wait for the judge to take down his notes either on paper or, increasingly, on his laptop.

Giving evidence

Each witness in the court will give evidence in three parts. First, the examination-in-chief takes place, when the side that has called you will ask questions about your examination, having established who you are and what are your qualifications and relevant experience.

Ask the judge's permission to refer to your contemporaneous notes. They may already have been seen by the prosecution and served on the defence. If not, be prepared to hand them over during your evidence.

Leading questions, i.e. those that suggest the answer, are not allowed unless agreed by the judge and both counsel. It is not uncommon for that to be agreed and for the witness to be led through undisputed parts of the evidence. For example, "You saw Joan Smith on 30th June last year did you not? This was at the request of D.C. Brown and took place at a specially designated suite?".

You will then be asked to describe your findings. Counsel may want to deal with specific relevant injuries, such as marks on the neck consistent with attempted strangulation or the genital injuries, or they may ask you to give a general account for the jury of what you found.

You should describe the injuries in a logical sequence. I usually start with the head and work down, following the order in which I would normally do the examination, using medical terms explained to the jury in lay terms, for example, an abrasion is a scratch.

Copies of your body charts are usually circulated to lawyers and jury and it is helpful to point out on your own person (the top half at any rate) where the injuries were.

You will then be asked for your opinion as to what caused the injuries and, again, it is useful to show the jury, for example by gripping your own arm, how the injury might have been caused.

The cross-examination

After the Prosecution barrister has finished his examination he will say, "Please wait there," and the defence barrister will rise to his feet.

This is quite a dramatic moment because you never know what is coming next. The defence barrister will want to pick up on any discrepancy between your witness statement and your oral evidence. He will want to put it to you that there are other explanations for the injuries that you have described. A good barrister will have formed a clear assessment of you as a witness during your examination-in-chief and will tailor his strategy accordingly.

If your evidence has been well presented, objective and unbiased, there may be little or no cross-examination. If you have been too dogmatic in your examination-in-chief, counsel may suggest that you are biased in favour of the prosecution. He may then want to go into your background and qualifications and may make a point such as, "You only do examinations of victims and only appear for the prosecution"; "You work for or are paid by the police", suggesting bias. The way to deal with this is to stand on your dignity and say that you are an independent professional and are paid out of public funds, adding if you like, "as is everyone in this court", but do not be arrogant. You do not want to annoy the judge or jury.

"It's not the art of examining crossly it's the art of leading the witness through a line of proposition he agrees to until he is forced to agree to the one fatal question."[3]

Cross-examination has also been described as "the greatest legal engine ever invented for the discovery of truth" and "one of the most base and depraved of all possible employment of intellectual power".[4]

A good cross-examination is rather like a game of chess, with counsel knowing exactly what his object is and where he is going. He may put a series of questions about a particular topic and then leave that topic apparently unfinished but with a piece strategically placed on the board. After pursuing another line of questioning, gaining minor adjustments of the evidence, he will then return to his previous subject and hope to show that the witness's answers are inconsistent. "A general conclusion which the witness would not accept at first, may be reached indirectly e.g. by building it up from specific points or by combining separate facts to give that result."[4]

It is of vital importance for the witness to try and understand where the cross-examination is leading and, if possible, to be able to think of the next question but one (or two or three) and not allow counsel to take you along that road. You can only really do that if you have done your homework the night before.

Hypothetical questions may be put to you. If you answer them without qualification you may be being led along a path that will discredit your evidence. For example, you might be asked to agree that a rape complainant would be very distressed. Experienced doctors know that rape complainants may be very quiet and cooperative and not overtly distressed. You should be careful not to agree and may suggest that you should explain to the jury in more detail why you cannot agree.

Many doctors find cross-examination stressful and irritating, perhaps because they are not used to having their opinions questioned. However, coping with a well-prepared cross-examination by a good barrister can be a stimulating and rewarding experience. Be prepared to concede where reasonable but stick on points which you feel that the court should rely upon. Do not step outside your own field of expertise and resist any temptation from counsel to do so.

The re-examination

Following the cross-examination, the prosecuting barrister is allowed to re-examine. This is to clarify any points that have been muddied by the defence and perhaps to try to win back some lost ground. There can be no leading questions and no new subjects can be put.

THE BOTTOM LINE

Remember:

- Rape is not a medical diagnosis, it is a legal concept.
- You have only a keyhole view into a situation where there may be honest differences as to what took place.
- Do not say things in court that you would not say in front of your peers.
- Do not give opinions that could properly be within the remit of the jury from their own experience.
- Do not allow counsel to pick off injuries one by one; look at the whole picture, but do not try to add in, for example, all the bruises, some of which may be weeks old.
- If you make a mistake, admit it.
- If new information is put to you, consider it carefully and concede where appropriate.

The defence medical expert

These days it is the norm for the defendant's solicitor to instruct a defence medical expert. While some doctors may find it threatening to have their opinion challenged, my view is that this is in the interests of justice and that honest and reliable evidence may be strengthened by being scrutinised by another expert.

A defence expert is not there to enable rapists to walk free, any more than the prosecution's doctor is there to secure a conviction. They are there to assist in the administration of justice in seeing that verdicts are based on sound evidence that can withstand challenge.

The defence doctor will receive a large bundle of papers in the case, including the witness statement of the complainant, all the medical evidence, the transcript of the tape recorded interviews of the defendant and his defence statement in which he sets out his view of events. It is vitally important that the defence doctor sees the contemporaneous medical notes of the examination.

It is not rare for there to be discrepancies between the notes and the witness statement; for example, in two cases in which I was involved injuries described in witness statements as being in the vulva were clearly shown on the body charts in the medical notes as being in the groin.

In another of my cases, an important point crucial to the case arose where samples 1, 2, 3 and 4 taken by the doctor who examined the defendant had not been submitted for forensic analysis, even though the other specimens had been. They were swabs taken from a possible suction bruise ('love bite') on the complainant's neck and were important evidence supporting the defendant's account of events. The doctor instructed by the defence was able to bring this to the attention of the court and after the complainant's evidence proved to be very unreliable, the judge directed the jury to acquit.

The doctor instructed by the defence will usually sit in court throughout the prosecution case and will advise counsel during the medical evidence. It can be quite daunting to see a well-known member of the profession passing notes to counsel during your evidence. Counsel will sometimes ask their expert to be in court because they feel that the medical evidence will be more balanced if it is given in the presence of another doctor. The defence medical expert is commonly not called to give evidence if the cross-examination has achieved its objective.

The defence doctor's report may:

- cause the defendant to plead guilty when he realises the strength of the evidence against him
- cause the CPS to drop the case or substitute a lesser charge, e.g. indecent assault instead of rape
- provide points for counsel for cross-examination.

Dilemmas

Medical evidence, in criminal cases, is of variable quality with some doctors being well trained and experienced and others lacking appropriate skills. Doctors who only examine a few complainants and who have no training in forensic medicine may not be capable of providing the quality of evidence which the courts expect and some defence experts also lack the necessary experience and training.

The doctor carrying out the initial examination of the complainant has limited knowledge of the facts and sometimes may stick dogmatically to an opinion formed on inadequate information and not be prepared to modify that opinion in the light of further knowledge.

There have been instances where, had the doctor obtained all the information that was available, it would have been obvious that the medical findings were not consistent with the history given; for example, a child who said she was assaulted at about 11 o'clock in the morning by a family member would not start to bleed after going to pass a large hard stool at 7 o'clock in the evening. In that case, the child had been repeatedly questioned by the mother as to whether grandfather had abused her, when in fact the bleeding had been caused by an innocently sustained anal fissure.

What is relevant?

There is still uncertainty as to the amount of information that should be recorded by the examining doctor, who decides at the time of the examination what is and is not relevant. If details are omitted from the record then the doctor can clearly be accused of bias but the recording of full details of past psychiatric or gynaecological problems may not be in a complainant's best interest nor assist the administration of justice and has been criticised by lawyers.[5]

Criticism of examination techniques

Defence doctors sometimes have a tendency to criticise an examination that has not been as thorough as a full gynaecological examination. However, the doctor conducting the examination must behave with sensitivity and understanding and only do what is possible and relevant. It is vital that the examination itself is not perceived by the complainant as an assault. The doctor who has not, for instance, been able to insert a speculum into the vagina because of the age of the complainant or her reluctance to consent to the examination should not accept a defence expert's opinion that it was incompetent not to carry out such a procedure.

The training of doctors

Doctors carrying out rape examinations who are not fully trained in this area sometimes give inaccurate accounts of injuries, confusing lacerations caused by blunt trauma with incised wounds caused by sharp objects or suggesting that abrasions or lacerations could have been caused weeks earlier when the natural history of such injuries is that they heal in a matter of days. It is fairly well recognised now that giving an opinion on the age of bruises is likely to be inaccurate at best. However, firm evidence with regard to the healing of other injuries is lacking.

Dealing with the defence report

The first time you receive a defence medical expert report you may be quite daunted. It will look impressive, with details of the author's curriculum vitae, and may run to many pages. Much of that will be reiterating the details of the case and providing background information. Some doctors regularly engaged in defence work use the same paragraphs in almost every report they write. There are likely to be only two or three paragraphs that may be of real importance to the case and there may be no major difference between the doctors.

A written response should be provided for the CPS on receipt of the defence medical report, which you have insisted upon seeing the week before the trial.

A problem arises here because the examining doctor has not usually seen the witness statement of the complainant but will only have the account given by the police officer and, briefly, by the complainant at the time of the examination. If there is any doubt in your mind as to the degree of violence alleged to have been used, then you should ask the CPS to provide you with the complainant's statement before you prepare your response.

In the past, professional witnesses were never allowed to see other evidence in the case, for fear of the witness being influenced by it to alter their own evidence. The professional witness is not normally permitted to sit in court during the evidence of other witnesses. However, where you are providing an expert opinion on another expert's opinion, the court should recognise you as an expert, allow you to sit in court throughout the case, if necessary, and remunerate appropriately.

Where a doctor is relatively inexperienced, it is becoming more common for the CPS to instruct a more experienced doctor who may be able to deal more effectively with the defence medical expert. This is likely to become more widely used in the future and will improve the quality and reliability of medical evidence. Even if this is not the case, an inexperienced doctor should seek the advice of senior colleagues before responding to the defence report.

The myths of rape

The myths of rape – that an innocent virgin is attacked by a stranger, outside, sustains dramatic injuries and reports immediately to the police – are, unfortunately, still widely held by members of the public, including juries, and by some lawyers. In many of the cases where I receive instructions from solicitors, the assumption appears to be that rape could not have occurred without considerably more in the way of injuries than had been sustained. As the incidence of reported rape has risen, more women raped by a person known to them have come forward and, in many cases, the issue is purely one of consent.

In such cases, there may well be little, if any, genital or other injury and the honest expert opinion of the doctor instructed by the defence that injuries are seen in only a minority of cases of alleged rape will be of great assistance to defence lawyers, enabling them to understand more clearly the likely issues on which the trial will be decided.

Many reports prepared by doctors instructed by the defence will not be served on the prosecution, whereas in a civil case where the court authorises the instruction of the expert, the report will always be disclosed.

Some defence doctors provide reports and give evidence, saying that there would have been bruises or other injuries if the allegations made by the complainant were correct. It is perfectly fair to suggest that there might well have been injuries, but not to say that these would certainly have occurred if the complainant's account of events were true. A doctor making such a statement on behalf of the defence should be vigorously challenged by the prosecution doctor, referring to published literature on the incidence of injuries in cases of alleged rape. Perhaps some of these doctors are them-selves guilty of believing the myths of rape.

The incidence of injuries

The fact is that we do not know the incidence of genital injuries in consensual acts and it does not assist the jury for a doctor to state dogmatically that the injuries could not have been caused during consensual activity because no-one would consent to the acts alleged. This is clearly a matter for the jury and not for the, perhaps, rather naive doctor. There is a dearth of published work on this subject and considerable concern about the reliability and validity of the articles which are sometimes quoted.

It is within the experience of most gynaecologists that dramatic genital injuries can be sustained during consensual acts and these do not only occur on first sexual intercourse. It is important for the doctor to concede, where reasonably appropriate, that the findings, both general physical injuries and genital injuries, may have another innocent explanation, but it is perfectly proper to say "That is possible, but not in the least likely".

The credibility of a witness depends upon:

- training and experience
- knowledge of current thinking
- objectivity and lack of bias
- ability to communicate.

Some of the problems for doctors in court include:

- failure to communicate to the people who matter, i.e. the judge and jury
- use of medical jargon, not explained in lay terms
- arrogance
- failing to listen carefully to the question and perhaps answering a different question from the one put
- offering too much information.

Finally, in carrying out rape examinations and being prepared to give evidence in court, you are providing a valuable service to the community. It is stressful, with its unsocial hours, difficulties in fitting in court appearances with your other professional work and the hazards of the court itself. However, if you can cope, it can be an enormously rewarding professional experience and if you manage to get the better of a Queen's Counsel and cause him to sit down and end his cross-examination because you knew much more about the subject than he did, that will make up for the time when you misread right and left on your body charts when preparing your statement and had to admit that in court.

References

1.   A Review of the Criminal Courts of England and Wales by The Right Honourable Lord Justice Auld. Criminal Courts Review, September 2001. [www.criminal-courts-

review.org.uk/] Accessed 2 September 2003.

2. Saukko P, Knight B. *Knight's Forensic Pathology*. 3rd ed. Oxford: Oxford University Press; 2004.

3. Mortimer J. *Clinging to the Wreckage: A Part of Life*. London: Viking Press; 1987.

4. Stone M. *Cross Examination in Criminal Trials*. London: Butterworth; 1998.

5. Temkin J. Medical evidence in rape cases: a continuing problem for criminal justice. *Modern Law Review* 1998;61:821–48.

Chapter 12

Supporting the victim

Helen Reeves and Kate Mulley

Introduction

The impact of rape cannot be underestimated. It can reach out to touch every aspect of a person's life: their health, personal relationships and financial security. It can affect where and with whom a person wishes to live, their perception of themselves and of the world.

Last year, Victim Support offered help to just under 20 000 people who had become the victims of rape or other sexual crime. While these people's lives may never be the same again, all the evidence suggests that being treated sympathetically and being provided with support can make a real difference to long-term recovery. The message is clear: victims of sexual violence need to be safe, they need to be believed and they need to be treated with respect.

This chapter provides an insight into some of the issues faced by women who have been raped and then considers what help is available and the ways in which this help can be accessed. The dilemmas section looks at how the actions of the different agencies and professions with whom women come into contact can impact on their recovery, either assisting or hindering the healing process.

Prevalence and impact

"At the time I couldn't imagine anything more horrifying than the prospect of dying, of being murdered. I realise now that surviving the attack was instinct. Surviving life after the attack is quite a different thing."

According to Home Office statistics, 37,300 sexual offences were recorded by the police in 2000/01.[1] Although overall figures for sexual offences fell slightly from previous years, there was a 2% increase in the number of recorded rapes to 8600. These official crime statistics include the 654 cases of male rape that were reported to the police. Victim Support offers practical help and information to men who have been raped or sexually assaulted. However, as the focus of this book is on women, the remainder of this chapter focuses exclusively on female victims.

The vast majority of crimes of sexual violence are never reported to the police: various surveys suggest that between 75% and 90% of all rapes go unreported. Women may decide not to report the offence for a variety of reasons: because they knew their attacker, fear of reprisal or because of the likely reactions of their family. Some women will not realise that the abuse they have suffered is a criminal offence, particularly if it occurs within a relationship. In addition, reporting is likely to be influenced by perceptions of a criminal justice system that is perceived as unsympathetic to the needs of victims and rarely convicts on a charge of rape.

So who are the victims? Just as there is no typical rapist, nor is there a 'typical' rape victim. Although most women who are raped are young adults, young children, pregnant mothers and elderly women are also raped. The majority of rapes take place indoors and are committed by someone known to the victim.

~ Women have different ways of responding to and coping with sexual violence. In 2001/02, 4965 rape victims were referred to Victim Support.[2] Some of the more common reactions these women have described include feeling frightened, guilty, powerless, angry, ashamed and depressed, and having difficulty eating, sleeping or concentrating. Many women feel that they have lost control of their lives and that their self-esteem has been undermined. If their partner is the offender, the impact may be even greater. In addition, the links between sexual and domestic violence have been well established, so that for some women sexual violence is not a one-off event but a continuing experience. Many women make a full recovery but some will be seriously affected in the longer term. These women are sometimes described as suffering from post-traumatic stress disorder. This syndrome describes a pattern of symptoms, some or all of which may be experienced, which include violent nightmares, intrusive thoughts of the event or flash-backs, numbing, avoidance and feelings of arousal, confusion or emptiness.

A woman's ability to cope with the trauma of being raped will be affected by the real or imagined reactions of her partner, her family or friends. She may feel that she is partly or totally to blame for the incident and so be reluctant to expose herself to the criticism and harsh judgement of others. In addition, many women feel guilty about burdening their family and friends and causing them distress by talking about the crime. People may not be as supportive as she would wish. Sometimes people feel a need to distance themselves from the crime, urging the victim to put it behind them. Often people just do not know what to say and so avoid the subject.

Because of the overwhelming psychological impact of rape, sometimes the practical effects can be overlooked. Being raped can affect an individual's ability to live her daily life. Some women are unable to return to work, others feel unable to be on their own or, if the attack took place at home, cannot face going home at all. If a child is born as a result of the attack, the long-term costs of looking after the child will only partly be met by social security. Women who have been raped and who have reported the offence to the police can submit a claim to the Criminal Injuries Compensation Authority.

However, it can take months or even years before claims are granted. In addition, awards for psychological injury (as opposed to physical injury) are relatively low and the compensation authority has adopted a narrow definition of sexual crime.

Provision of support

"Get angry and get support. Get whatever it takes to make you feel good about yourself again."

Immediately after an attack, the woman's safety must be the first priority. In the longer term, how a woman reacts and her recovery will depend on an infinite number of factors, not least her personality or life experiences. Women who receive a sympathetic hearing are at an advantage over those who are blamed for the offence. Being able to share and validate your feelings can make a real difference to the recovery process.

Women who have been raped or sexually assaulted have a range of different needs. They may have urgent medical needs or require specialist medical intervention to assist their long-term recovery. They may wish to talk in confidence with someone outside their normal social circle. They may need information, for example about any criminal process or about practical issues such as personal security or compensation. They may need an advocate to help them in their dealings with other agencies, such as housing authorities or the police. Women may need help with an emergency move to secure accommodation or a refuge. They may also want to meet and talk with other women who have suffered similar experiences.

A variety of national and local voluntary agencies provide specialist services to women who have been raped or sexually assaulted, the best known of which are Victim Support, Rape Crisis and Women's Aid. Rape Crisis groups offer free and confidential counselling and support to women and girl survivors of rape and sexual abuse. Women's Aid is the national charity working to end domestic violence against women and children. Their mission is to advocate for abused women and children and to offer support and a place of safety by providing refuges and other services. There are also a number of local groups, including self-help groups or services for particular groups of women. The remainder of this section looks at the services provided by Victim Support and the Witness Service and then considers how agencies can work together to help women who have been raped or sexually assaulted.

Victim Support

"It was important to have someone outside of my family and friends that I could talk to."

Victim Support is the national charity that helps people to cope with crime. Each year, trained staff and volunteers offer emotional support, practical help and information to over one million people who have suffered crimes such as burglary, sexual assault, racial violence, theft or even the violent death of a loved one. Sadly, the demand for services rises every year and the number of people turning to Victim Support following crimes of violence, sexual assault and murder is increasing dramatically.

Victim Support provides a specialist service for women who have been raped or sexually assaulted that is run to national standards and covers the whole country. All Victim Support volunteers and staff who provide this service have been specially selected and must have successfully completed our specialist-training programme. A female volunteer or member of staff must always make contact with women who have been raped or sexually assaulted.

Victim Support can help women who have been raped or sexually assaulted by:

- listening to women and allowing them time to talk about their feelings
- helping people to talk through issues relating to the crime; for example, whether or not to report it to the police or to tell family members
- providing information about any urgent practical, medical and personal safety issues that may arise and about any criminal proceedings
- providing advocacy with other agencies or individuals
- accompanying women to the police station or to court, etc.
- providing practical help, such as filling in forms or writing letters
- visiting women in their own homes or, if more appropriate, arranging to see them elsewhere
- referring women to other agencies where appropriate (with the woman's consent)
- giving information about compensation and helping with applications.

There is no time limit on service provision from Victim Support and a separate service can also be provided to other family members.

Victim Support's services are free and confidential. The organisation respects the individual's autonomy to make her own decisions, with the aim of helping women to regain control of their lives. The organisation believes that it is their role to make their services accessible but not to tell people what they need or should do.

Most of the women who take up the service have been told about Victim Support by the police, who will have asked them if they would like to be referred to the service. Women who have not reported the crime can contact Victim Support directly, either by contacting their local Victim Support service or by calling the Victim Supportline. However, at the moment only a relatively low percentage of total referrals come through the support line and there are only limited resources to promote this service.

Victim Support provides services for victims of domestic violence, working with other local agencies to ensure the best use of resources. Examples of other agencies that Victim Support can liaise with for the benefit of the victim are Women's Aid, Homestart, Well Women Centres, Sure Start, Citizen's Advice Bureaux, local council housing departments, Child and Family Support Services, Young Concern, local counselling services, drug and alcohol centres, legal advice, local and national refuges, rape and sexual abuse services plus many more. All Victim Support volunteers receive awareness training about the impact of domestic violence, which is vital as they provide an outreach service, meaning that some individuals will reveal domestic violence where they have not felt able to disclose this before. Many Victim Support services also undertake long-term work with victims of domestic violence and volunteers are trained specifically for this work. We offer emotional support and explore options with people in a safe place. We help people to attend meetings, apply for criminal injuries compensation and support them in court if they choose to pursue their case. It is our policy not to replicate services, but rather to work in partnership with other agencies. We are proactive in helping people to access services that can help by referral or by sign-posting them, for example to legal advisors, Women's Aid, Refuge, housing and benefits agencies.

For the few cases that do go to court, Victim Support's Witness Service is available. Going to court and giving evidence can be a confusing and distressing experience for all witnesses and these feelings are likely to be exacerbated for rape victims, especially if they know their attacker or where consent is an issue. The Witness Service, now running in all criminal courts in England and Wales, offers information and emotional support to witnesses before, during and after hearings. It can arrange pre-court familiarisation visits to show witnesses around an empty courtroom and to explain procedures and the roles of court personnel. The Witness Service also provides private waiting areas at court, to ensure that victims and witnesses do not have to sit near the defendant or their family. Volunteers can accompany witnesses into court when they are called to give evidence and are available afterwards to talk through the experience. They can also put witnesses in touch with other help, including their local Victim Support service.

"I believed the trial would make everything OK and that I would be able to get back to normal, but afterwards I had this hollow feeling. Everyone else thought it was all over, only Victim Support didn't disappear when everyone else did."

Victim Support also contributes to interagency partnerships such as domestic violence forums. In some parts of the country multi-agency projects have been set up specifically for women who have been raped or sexually assaulted. The value of these projects is in ensuring that all the relevant services are available to women under one roof, including facilities for reporting and the forensic examination, as well as help with medical issues and referral on for continuing support. Victim Support services link into these projects to ensure that women receive as seamless a service as possible.

The dilemmas

Specialist support services are available to women who have been raped or sexually assaulted. However, on their own, these services will never be sufficient. Women who have been raped will come into contact with a variety of different agencies both within the community and, if they choose to report the offence, in the criminal justice system. The response of these agencies is crucial. First, they need to know what help is available and pass this information on to victims, and second, they need to ensure that their own response is appropriate and not likely to exacerbate the woman's distress.

Community response

As has already been said, the vast majority of crimes of sexual violence are not reported to the police. Many women will never speak about the offence but others may disclose what has happened to a variety of different local agencies or professionals. It is important that all the agencies with whom women come into contact are aware of the support that is available. Victim Support aims to publicise its services as widely as possible both nationally, through national campaigns and media coverage, and locally, through local media or by placing leaflets in doctor's surgeries, accident and emergency departments, public libraries, community halls, etc. However, it is a voluntary organisation and the budget for this type of promotional work is limited.

Victims of crime are more likely to contact healthcare workers than any other professional. This may be for a variety of reasons: if they were injured in the attack; testing for pregnancy or sexually transmitted diseases, including HIV; or if they are suffering from depression or would like a referral for counselling or psychiatric help. Victim Support's report *Criminal Neglect: No Justice Beyond Criminal Justice*[3] highlighted health as a specific area of need for crime victims. Particular problems include: widely differing levels of awareness; services being organised and accessed differently in different parts of the country; and varying levels of service provision.

"I was asked if I wanted to see a counsellor. But because it was so far away, and I am now registered blind, there is no way I could have got there. I hardly ever go out of the house now, only to the corner shop."

Access to and availability of counselling services varies greatly across the country, which leads to lengthy waiting times. Victim Support believes that people who have been the victims of crime should not have to pay for the services they need simply to get help more quickly. In addition, victims of crime should not have to pay for medical documentation or certificates (i.e. letters in support of rehousing, to take time off work, or to support claims for compensation.). In the *Criminal Neglect* report,[3] an integrated approach to meeting the healthcare needs of crime victims and for the drawing up of national standards is called for.

Similar problems exist in the housing sector and other areas of social provision. Public agencies need training to enable their personnel to recognise the emotional impact of crime. A coordinated response is necessary to avoid secondary victimisation and to ensure that victims are made aware of the types of help that are available.

Criminal justice

"The victim is made to feel guilty and victimised twice over: once with the incident and secondly with the treatment they receive from the courts."

A perception of the criminal justice system's unsympathetic treatment of victims, especially rape victims, is the reason some people choose not to report sexual offences. Those who do report often express a high degree of dissatisfaction; with Home Office research suggesting that as many as 33% of all witnesses would not be happy to be a witness again.[4]

As well as being a service provider, Victim Support works to increase understanding and awareness of the effects of crime and to ensure better recognition of victim's rights. Because of the extent of our contact with victims and witnesses, they are in a unique position to gather information about the impact of crime. They are also able to monitor the introduction of changes to the criminal justice system, examining how they are perceived and used by victims.

In 1996, Victim Support published: *Women, Rape and the Criminal Justice System*.[5] The report looked at the experiences of over 1000 women who reported rape and highlighted the problems they faced during the criminal justice process. The report identified three main areas of concern:

- lack of information
- the need for protection in the community
- the way women are treated at court when they are called to give evidence (particularly during the cross-examination).

Several new measures have appeared aiming to improve the treatment of witnesses, some of which apply specifically to victims of sexual violence. Various agencies working within criminal justice now have duties relating victims and witnesses: the Crown Prosecution Service will have responsibility for ensuring that victims are informed of key decisions in their case and the Probation Service has new responsibilities for contact with a number of victims whose offenders are in prison. Victim personal statements have been introduced for cases going through the courts to enable victims to communicate any particular needs or concerns they may have and for these to be taken into account, for example in bail decisions etc.

"I feel that victims are not represented in court. The control that is taken away from you when you are raped is repeated."

In 1998, the Home Office published the *Speaking Up for Justice* report.[6] This report recommended extensive new measures to improve the treatment of vulnerable and intimidated witnesses, including a range of special measures that were incorporated in the Youth Justice and Criminal Evidence Act 1999. The special measures include the screening of witnesses from defendants, provisions for witnesses to give evidence by live television link or in private, i.e. clearing the courtroom. There is a presumption that victims of rape and some other sexual offences will automatically qualify for special measures, if they wish. The Act also introduced provisions in rape trials to restrict the circumstances in which evidence or questions about a complainant's sexual behaviour outside the circumstances of the alleged offence can be introduced. It also changed the law regarding cross-examination by the defendant in person.

In July 2000, the Home Office published *Setting the Boundaries: Reforming the Law on Sexual Offences.*[7] This report called for a redefinition of the laws on rape and sexual assault and took the view that the judgement of right and wrong should be based on an assessment of the harm done to the individual.

Then, in April 2002, HM Crown Prosecution Service Inspectorate (CPSI) and HM Inspectorate of Constabulary published a report on the joint inspection into investigation and prosecution of cases involving allegations of rape.[8] This report acknowledges that there are few offences that impact so severely on the victim as rape and the report made several recommendations which include:

- an immediate review by all police forces of the facilities for victim examination
- a review by the Association of Chief Police Officers of the role of the forensic medical examiner including training and recruitment of female examiners
- a review of the training of police officers who deal with rape victims
- allocation of rape cases to specialist lawyers, and ensuring all major review decisions are subject to discussion with a second specialist
- ensuring that instructions are given to challenge offensive and seemingly irrelevant questioning in court.

This report was followed up in July 2002 by an action plan to implement the recommendations of the joint inspection.[9]

It does appear that the Government and the professionals working within criminal justice are taking action through legislation to improve the process for victims of sexual violence. These provisions have still to be successfully implemented and all the agencies responsible for their implementation will need to receive training for this role. Yet, within this flurry of activity, some problems remain outstanding, despite recommendations for change such as facilities for the medical examination, the disclosure of medical records and the process of cross-examination.

Medical examination

"I walked into this room and this lady came up to me and said 'Oh my God, what has he done to you?' It was wonderful. I wish everyone could have had her – how could they use male doctors?"

Victim Support's report *Women, Rape and the Criminal Justice System*[5] showed that seeing a sympathetic female forensic medical examiner in a specially designed rape examination suite can dramatically improve what is essentially a traumatic experience. The majority of the women interviewed for the report did not have these facilities.

There is also a concern that, although the function of forensic medical examiners is not to provide continuing medical help, they should ensure that women are aware of the issues and are referred on. The examiner should advise the woman to consult her own GP or to make an appointment at her local hospital's genitourinary clinic, where the appropriate tests can be made and specialist counselling is usually available. They could also act as a point of referral to other services, such as Victim Support. The setting up of specially designed centres, which bring the various different agencies together in a holistic way, provides a model for the future.

"The medical should be made easier and you should be prepared for what they do to you. He (the doctor) didn't tell me what he was going to do next. You feel like a nonentity sometimes – some things were so embarrassing. I was crying and it was so cold in there."

Pre-trial therapy and the use of medical records

"I was on trial, not him, without a doubt."

Victim Support believes that victims and witnesses should have access to therapy if they need it and that there should be a presumption that therapy will only rarely be relevant to the criminal case. This means a therapist should be able to assure their client confidentiality. No criminal justice agency should have the right to know that therapy is proposed, being undertaken or has been undertaken. Only a court should have the power to decide what information is relevant and therefore what must be disclosed, and the victim or witness should always be informed of any request for or granting of disclosure. At the moment, women do not have these guarantees, which means that either they may delay or abandon seeking the help they require or that personal, and often irrelevant, material is routinely dragged into the court process.

The cross-examination

"It was a historical and political battle between the ego's of two barristers – and I was the victim."

The aspect of the trial that evokes the greatest criticism is the way in which witnesses, particularly those for the prosecution, are cross-examined after giving their evidence. This issue has been raised in successive government reports, such as Lord Justice Auld's *Review of the Criminal Courts*[10] and the *Speaking Up for Justice* report.[6] Recommendations for action are contained within the CPSI thematic review into the prosecution of cases involving allegations of rape. It seems that, although there is general agreement that more control needs to be exercised in the interests of justice, there is continuing concern, particularly among the legal professions, about the means by which improvements can be achieved.

A particular issue for many rape trials is the admission of questions on the complainant's previous sexual history. The law in this area has now been changed for a second time. The Youth Justice and Criminal Evidence Act 1999 states that, where the issue is one of consent, evidence of previous sexual behaviour can only be permitted where the behaviour happened at or about the same time as the alleged rape or was so similar to the behaviour at the time of the alleged offence that it could not be explained as coincidence. However, this section of the Act has now been challenged under the Human Rights Act 1998. In May 2001, a case in the House of Lords held that excluding evidence of a previous sexual relationship between the complainant and the defendant altogether could breach the defendant's right to a fair trial.[11] The Law Lords ruled that the law must be read so as to make it compatible with the Human Rights Act, restoring trial judges some of the discretion removed by Section 41 of the Youth Justice and Criminal Evidence Act. In future, the trial judges must decide whether the evidence the defendant wants to put forward is relevant to the issue of whether or not the complainant consented to sex on the occasion in question. If so, the evidence will be allowed. Research is being undertaken on behalf of the Home Office to investigate the use of Section 41 and the results of this research will prompt further action to ensure that inappropriate questioning of rape complainants does not take place.

Conclusion

Currently, more women are reporting rape than ever before and yet there has been a steady decrease in the rate of convictions. New initiatives are being introduced but it remains to be seen whether there is the necessary will to take these reforms further and to tackle some of the most persistently difficult issues. The major new initiatives for vulnerable witnesses and the reform of the law on sex offences have yet to be introduced. It is to be hoped that they will make a real difference to women's experiences of the criminal justice process and to public perceptions of the system.

Yet, even if the criminal justice system becomes drastically more sensitive, many women will still never choose to make a formal complaint of rape, often for good reasons. Just because women have not reported a sexual offence does not mean they do not need support. Frequently, the opposite is the case. It is the duty of all the various agencies with whom women come into contact to make sure that their staff are trained and able to provide an appropriate response, and that they are aware of the range of support which is available to the victims of sexual violence in the community.

References

1. Home Office. *Criminal Statistics: England and Wales 2000: Statistics Relating to Crime and Criminal Proceedings for the Year 2000. Presented to Parliament by the Secretary of State for the Home Department by Command of Her Majesty December 2001.* Cm 5312. London: Stationery Office; 20001. [www.archive.official-documents.co.uk/document/cm53/5312/crimestats.pdf] Accessed 2 September 2003.
2. Victim Support. *Annual Report and Accounts for the year ended 31 March 2002 With Statistical Appendix 31 March 2002.* London: Victim Support; 2002. [www.victimsupport.org.uk/about/publications/annual_report/accounts_2002.pdf] Accessed 2 September 2003.
3. Victim Support. *Criminal Neglect: No Justice Beyond Criminal Justice.* London: Victim Support; February 2002. [www.victimsupport.org.uk/about/publications/neglect/criminal_neglect.html] Accessed 2 September 2003.
4. Angle H, Malam S, Carey C. *Witness Satisfaction: Findings from the Witness Satisfaction Survey 2002.* Home Office Research and Statistics Directorate. Research Findings No 189. London: Home Office; 2003 [www.homeoffice.gov.uk/rds/pdfs2/rdsolr1903.pdf].
5. Victim Support. *Women, Rape and the Criminal Justice System.* London: Home Office; 1996.
6. Home Office. *Speaking Up for Justice: Report of the Interdepartmental Working Group on the Treatment of Vulnerable or Intimidated Witnesses in the Criminal Justice System.* London: Home Office; June 1998. [www.homeoffice.gov.uk/docs/sufj.pdf] Accessed 2 September 2003.
7. Home Office. *Setting the Boundaries: Reforming the Law on Sex Offences.* London: Home Office Communication Directorate; July 2000.
8. HM Crown Prosecution Service Inspectorate and HM Inspectorate of Constabulary. *A Report on the Joint Inspection into the Investigation and Prosecution of Cases Involving Allegations of Rape.* London: Home Office; April 2002 [www.homeoffice.gov.uk/hmic/CPSI_HMIC_Rape_Thematic.pdf].
9 Home Office, Court Service, Crown Prosecution Service. Action plan to implement the recommendations of the HMCPSI/HMIC joint investigation into the investigation and prosecution of cases involving allegations of rape. London: Home Office; July 2002 [www.homeoffice.gov.uk/docs/action_plan.pdf]. Accessed 8 April 2004.

10. A Review of the Criminal Courts of England and Wales by The Right Honourable Lord Justice Auld. Criminal Courts Review, September 2001. [www.criminal-courts-review.org.uk/] Accessed 2 September 2003.
11. RvA (2001) UKHL 25.

SECTION TWO
Domestic violence: the overlap with rape

Chapter 13

The impact of domestic violence in obstetrics

Helen Cameron

Introduction

Violence may be a more common problem for pregnant women than some conditions for which they are routinely screened and evaluated, and there is a growing body of evidence that shows that violent deaths among women are often associated with pregnancy events. The period of pregnancy presents a unique opportunity when clinicians and midwives have regular contact with women and this prenatal contact may allow the development of a relationship, which facilitates the disclosure of domestic violence. Domestic violence is used by the perpetrator to acquire power and control through instilling feelings of fear and insecurity and during pregnancy women are most vulnerable and least able to defend themselves or take evasive action. Acts of brutality are frequently followed by expressions of contrition and remorse by the perpetrator who promises to change, never to hit her again and telling the woman how much he loves her. Although there may be trends of increased prevalence of domestic violence in certain socio-economic groups, women of all ages, income and ethnic backgrounds may be subject to domestic violence or sexual assault in pregnancy.

Prevalence of domestic violence in pregnancy

Estimates of violence in clinic attendees vary according to the screening methods used but are likely to be underestimates as women are generally reluctant to disclose such experience (Table 13.1).

Between 10.9% and 27.5% of antenatal clinic attendees report a history of domestic violence in the past. Hillard[1] found that 10.9% of 742 women interviewed indicated that they had been victims of domestic violence before the current pregnancy, Helton et al.[2] found 15% and Hedin et al.[3] 27.5% of 207 women. For women revealing abuse in the current pregnancy, Hedin et al.[3] found that 95% had been abused in the past and McFarlane et al.[4] found 51.8% of 199 women who reported abuse at some point in the past.

Table 13.1 Prevalence of domestic violence in pregnancy

Authors	Reference	Year of publication	Women in study (*n*)	Prevalence (%)
Helton *et al.*	2	1987	290	8.0
Amaro *et al.*	43	1990	1243	7.0
O'Campo *et al.*	44	1994	358	65.0 (verbal and physical) 20.0 (moderate/severe)
Webster *et al.*	5	1994	1014	5.8 at booking 8.9 at 36 weeks
McFarlane *et al.*	20	1996	1203	16.0
Fernandez and Krueger	21	1999	489	20.0
Muhajarine and D'Arcy	45	1999	728	5.70
Martin	29	2001	2648	6.1
Johnson *et al.*	46	2003	475	17.0 at booking

Characteristics of domestic violence in pregnancy

Domestic violence may commence or escalate in pregnancy.[5] Hedin *et al.*[3] found that 4.3% of women had been exposed to serious violence in pregnancy and 3.3% to sexual violence. Recurrent abuse in pregnancy is common, with 60% of women disclosing abuse in pregnancy reporting two or three episodes of assault.[6] The bruising of physical abuse in pregnancy may be hidden and defensive marks on the forearms may be overlooked. The distribution of the injuries acquired in pregnancy is more likely on the breasts and abdomen than in nonpregnant victims and awareness that atypical marks on the abdomen may be a feature of abuse may help the clinician to identify more cases of undisclosed domestic violence. According to Hedin and Janson,[7] other frequent targets are the upper arms, forearms, face and neck.[8] This redirection of the assault implies hostility towards the woman's fertility.[9] From the Hedin and Janson study,[7] it was revealed that abused women in Sweden were significantly younger and single, and had lower income and education compared with non-abused women. This association between the increasing educational level of women and decrease in revealed abuse was also found in the Brisbane study.[5] It is possible that education moderates abusive behaviour or that educated women may feel more reluctant to admit their involvement in a violent relationship.

Women who experience physical violence are more likely to delay entry into prenatal care.[10]

In a stratified prospective cohort analysis of 1203 pregnant women in Texas, USA, McFarlane *et al.*[11] found that abused women were twice as likely to begin prenatal care during the third trimester, with abuse preceding late entry. The same group of researchers found that at interview, of 261 pregnant women who reported vaginal bleeding to an emergency department, 33.3% reported abuse.[12] The authors emphasised that abuse of pregnant women reporting to an emergency department was common. Traumatic placental abruption can occur as a direct result of blows inflicted to the abdomen and the clinician needs to be aware of the possibility of the victim giving a false history of how the injury had occurred.

Women who had experienced domestic violence in the current pregnancy were significantly more likely to have repeat admissions and those who reported having been victims of domestic violence in the 12 months prior to interview were significantly more likely to experience troublesome backache, headaches, hyperemesis or false labour.[13] Satin *et al.*[14] also found that sexually abused women had a higher incidence of multiple hospital admissions during pregnancy (15% versus 8%; $P < 0.01$) and emphasised that the opportunity for domestic violence screening should not be missed in such circumstances. Physical abuse is associated with significantly higher use of tobacco, alcohol and illicit drugs.[11,15]

Effect of age on prevalence of domestic violence

The prevalence of abuse among adolescents who are pregnant is even greater than for the adult pregnant women. Parker *et al.*[16] found that 21% of adolescents versus 14% of adult women reported violence during pregnancy. Webster *et al.*[5] also found that the prevalence of abuse during pregnancy decreased with increasing age with rates of 43.7% among the 103 teenagers in the Brisbane study, where the overall rate of abuse in pregnancy was 5.8%. Abused pregnant adolescents also appear to give birth to infants with significantly lower birthweights and have significantly more previous miscarriages.[17]

Domestic violence and pregnancy outcome

There are limited data on the perinatal effects of assault during pregnancy and thus there is a somewhat confused picture with no consistent patterns. Mezey and Bewley[13] found no significant association between domestic violence in the 12 months prior to interview and any experience of antenatal complications in the current pregnancy.

Low birth weight

Grimstad *et al.*[18] found that low birthweight was not associated with experience of any interpersonal conflict behaviour. The authors did not find any other pregnancy complications to be associated with abuse in pregnancy in the 84 women who delivered a low-birthweight infant compared with the 90 women who delivered a higher-birthweight baby. However, Campbell *et al.*[19] found that physical and nonphysical abuse were both significant risk factors for low birthweight for full-term but not preterm infants. The authors point out the importance of domestic violence screening at delivery, especially for women who may not have obtained prenatal care. More severe abuse was significantly correlated with low birthweight in a prospective study of 1203 women and abused white women delivered infants with the greatest reduction in birthweight.[20] Fernandez and Krueger[21] also found that domestic violence was a risk factor for low-birthweight babies and Renker[15] found that abused older adolescents were more likely to give birth to low-birthweight infants. The authors indicated that identification of abused adolescents may enhance prediction of infants at high risk and may provide opportunities for intervention. Although the incidence of low-birthweight infants, in a study of sexual assault victims by Satin et al.,[22] was 24% for assault patients versus 11%, he commented that without controlling for other factors such as drugs, alcohol and late prenatal care it remains unclear as to whether sexual assault increases the risk of low-birthweight infants or whether women at risk of having low-birthweight infants are more likely to be the victims of rape.

Preterm labour and delivery

Fernandez and Krueger[21] found that 22% of abused women had preterm deliveries compared with 6% in the control group ($P = 0.002$). Other studies also found that preterm labour strongly correlated with increasing acts of violence, with a 4.1-times greater risk of preterm labour in women who experienced severe violence as compared with those who experienced no maternal abuse.[23] Although Berenson et al.[16] found that women assaulted in the current pregnancy were twice as likely to require hospitalisation for treatment of preterm labour compared with those who denied assault, no difference was found in the prevalence of preterm delivery or low-birthweight babies.

Chorioamnionitis

Berenson et al.[16] demonstrated that assault victims were twice as likely to have chorioamnionitis as women who had not been abused but the small number of subjects in whom this complication developed prevented statistical procedures to control for confounders. Further prospective studies are required to evaluate the effects of domestic violence during pregnancy and the possible associations with adverse perinatal outcomes.

Miscarriage

With respect to risk of miscarriage, Jacoby et al.[24] found that young women who experienced abuse were substantially more likely to miscarry than their peers who had not been abused. However, Satin et al.[22] found that there were no spontaneous abortions within four weeks of the assault in a study of 114 pregnant assault victims.

Women with unwanted pregnancies

Pregnancy intendedness does appear to be associated with physical violence. Gazmararian et al.[25] found that women with unwanted pregnancies had 4.1 times the odds of experiencing physical violence than did women with intended pregnancies.

Using a self-administered five-question abuse assessment-screening tool together with one direct question regarding abuse as a factor in the abortion decision, Glander et al.[26] found that the prevalence of self-reported physical abuse was 39.5%.

Violence during the postpartum period

Psychosocial risk factors during the antenatal period may herald postpartum morbidity. In addition, violence may be more prevalent in the postpartum period than during pregnancy. In a study of 30 women with a history of abuse in pregnancy, there was a significant increase in the mean number of incidents of physical abuse per woman abused during the three months after delivery.[27] Gielen et al.[28] also reported that moderate to severe violence was more common during the postpartum period than prenatally. However, in the North Carolina Pregnancy Risk Assessment Monitoring System (NC PRAMS) it was found that less than 1% of all the 2648 respondents experienced abuse for the first time after infant delivery.[29] Reassuringly, the absence of any previous abuse was found to be strongly protective against postpartum abuse.

Rape-related pregnancy

In the USA, unintended pregnancy has been identified as a national epidemic and substantial resources have been dedicated to addressing this problem. To date, rape-related pregnancy has not been identified as a contributing factor in the unintended pregnancy rate. The risk of rape-related pregnancy has been estimated at approximately 5% of rape victims of reproductive age in the USA, where there are an estimated 32 101 pregnancies a year resulting from rape.[30] In Mexico, the rape-related pregnancy rate was estimated as 10%.[31] Of the 34 known cases of rape-related pregnancy in the previous study,[30] the majority occurred among adolescents and resulted from assault by a known, often related perpetrator.

In the USA, DNA typing has significantly altered the conviction rate but sometimes it is unclear from a victim's history whether a pregnancy has been achieved by the assailant or by a consensual partner. Resolution of pregnancy parentage in such circumstances may allow a couple to make an informed decision regarding continuation of the pregnancy. Blood can be taken from the woman and her consensual partner, and cultured amniotic or chorion villus cells can be submitted for fetal genetic analysis.[32] Paternity testing can thus positively exclude an alleged father or provide high likelihood of paternity.

Should a victim proceed with termination of a presumed rape-related pregnancy, abortion material can be submitted for genotyping. This can be undertaken immediately or the tissues can be stored for subsequent analysis.

Chorion villus sampling (CVS) provides an uncontaminated source of fetal tissue for genotyping compared with surgical abortion material, which consists of ruptured tissue of fetal and maternal origin. Undertaking CVS in such fraught circumstances may increase the victim's trauma but one could consider CVS under general anaesthetic immediately prior to the surgical termination of pregnancy. Medical termination of pregnancy might offer an alternative, less contaminated, source of fetal material.

Domestic violence and murder

As indicated in the Report on Confidential Enquiries into Maternal Deaths in United Kingdom 1997–1999, "Murder by a partner or ex-partner are at the extreme end of the spectrum of domestic violence".[33] Eight women were apparently murdered in such circumstances during the triennium and in all cases the all-too-obvious warning signs were present. In the USA, one-third of female homicides are committed by a present or former partner.[34] A follow-up of 41 injury-related maternal deaths in North Carolina, USA, revealed that 51.2% of these women were known to have or were suspected of having been abused, with the obstetric provider being at least suspicious of abuse in one-third of homicides committed by an intimate partner.[35]

Screening methods

Clinicians are taught that screening is undertaken on the basis that there is scientific evidence of effectiveness of screening and, thus, there should be an accurate test for the condition and also evidence that screening can prevent adverse health outcomes. Accordingly, this lack of evidence for effective interventions in domestic violence may serve as a disincentive for clinicians to ask about abuse. Indeed, guidelines from the National Institute for Clinical Excellence[36] state that there is insufficient evidence for the effectiveness of intervention in the healthcare setting for women identified by screening programmes. The guideline highlights the need for additional research to test the effectiveness of interventions on improving health outcomes before recommending routine screening. Healthcare professionals need to be alert to the symptoms and signs of domestic violence and women should be given the opportunity to disclose domestic violence in an environment in which they feel secure.

The use of a structured five-question screen was found to improve detection rates of battering both before and during pregnancy thus enabling clinicians a greater opportunity to intervene.[37] Included in the Norton questionnaire are questions about history of domestic violence, physical or sexual violence within the past year, violence during the current pregnancy, recent sexual abuse and fear of partner.

Asking women about violence at several points during their pregnancy may yield additional disclosure of domestic violence in women not previously recognised as abused.

The role of the health professional in recognising and responding to domestic violence is explored in more detail elsewhere in this volume and also in *Domestic Violence: A Resource Manual for Health Care Professionals*.[38]

Dilemmas in domestic violence

Prevalence estimation

The variation in the prevalence estimates depend upon factors that are both clinically and methodologically important. For example, the timing of screening for domestic violence in pregnancy may influence the prevalence rates; if screening is only undertaken in early pregnancy later abuse may be missed. The prevalence may be underestimated where women are only screened on admission for delivery, as women are under enormous stress at this time, especially if the partner is present. The number of times that women are screened for domestic violence in pregnancy may affect the prevalence, as may the characteristics of the inquiring health professional (professional category, race, gender or ethnic group). The form of the assessment is also important, i.e. whether it is a telephone enquiry, a self-administered questionnaire or a semi-structured interview. Each type of assessment has a different influence on the woman's perception of the degree of confidentiality, her trust in the process and the person undertaking the inquiry. Those who do not respond to inquiries form an important part of the overall picture, as illustrated by the NC PRAMS study, where the 25% of nonresponders were more likely to be young, unmarried, black and have lower educational attainment than the responders.[29]

Effects of domestic violence on breastfeeding

Little is known about domestic violence as a factor in the initiation or cessation of breastfeeding. It is possible that the abuser feels a sense of ownership of the woman's body. Within breastfeeding programmes, there should be a degree of sensitivity and awareness of the influence that domestic violence may have.

Domestic violence in pregnant adolescents

As the prevalence of domestic violence is even greater for adolescents than for adult women, programmes designed to deal with adolescent pregnancies need to address this problem in terms of prevention, early identification and specific interventions for this age group. Pregnant adolescents who are exposed to violence are at increased risk for substance abuse, inadequate prenatal care and poor birth outcome. After implementing a standardised screening tool for adolescents, Covington et al.[39] found a three-fold increase in the number reporting violence during their current pregnancy. The authors found that asking about specific behaviour such as hitting or kicking was more effective than using vague, loaded terms such violence or abuse. Larger studies in a broader context are needed to further address the issue of violence detection and domestic violence associations among the adolescent pregnant population. In the same way, further studies of cultural influences upon domestic violence need to be undertaken; it is simply not acceptable to put domestic violence down to 'cultural norms'.

Pregnancies in substance abusers

The interaction between domestic violence, substance abuse and pregnancy may be complex but there is a substantial body of evidence supporting links between pregnancy and substance abuse (including smoking and alcohol). As the triad of smoking, physical abuse and alcohol or illicit drugs are significantly related to infant birth weight there should be a systematic inclusion of screening and assessment for domestic violence where substance abuse is suspected.[11]

Confidentiality issues

Nationally, policies now exist that encourage partners to be present when women receive their maternity care and for women to carry their own maternity notes. This may impede the potential for women to seek help with domestic violence and also creates a challenge for health professionals to communicate details about abuse. Careful attention to confidentiality is needed to avoid putting women at risk.[40] As yet, there is no national guideline of best practice on ways of dealing with issues of confidentiality over domestic violence or substance abuse.

Intervention for domestic violence in pregnancy

Further research is also needed to investigate the benefits and cost of each component of interventions in pregnancy such as supporting and referring women who are identified as being at risk of, or experiencing domestic violence. So far, there is little evidence that intervention programmes affect actual pregnancy outcome but Parker et al.[41] did demonstrate that, regardless of age or ethnicity, basic information about abuse, resources and safety planning can affect positive outcomes for battered women in pregnancy when assessed six and twelve months post-intervention. A novel approach by

McFarlane and Wiist[42] involved the development of an advocacy model, evaluating the effectiveness of lay advocates ('Mentor Mothers') in establishing and maintaining contact with pregnant abused women throughout their pregnancy. Further studies are required to evaluate the outcomes related to this kind of intervention for domestic violence in pregnancy.

Conclusions

Armed with the knowledge of the prevalence of intimate partner abuse of women, the severity of abuse and its consequences for the pregnant woman and her infant and bearing in mind that the pregnant woman receives more frequent medical care than at any other time of her life, it becomes apparent that antenatal care provides a window of opportunity for screening, counselling and appropriate referral. If domestic violence screening is incorporated into antenatal care, assessment can serve as a primary health prevention measure for all women and as a secondary prevention measure for the abused woman. If pregnant women are not screened then domestic violence may remain undetected and this may place women at risk of domestic violence of escalating severity or even death. By raising awareness, undertaking domestic violence assessment, completing documentation and providing intervention measures routinely in antenatal care, clinicians have the opportunity to protect the vulnerable pregnant woman and her children and even to save their lives.

Further studies are still needed to evaluate the effects of domestic violence in pregnancy on measures of maternal health, fetal wellbeing and the obstetric outcome.

References

1. Hillard PJ. Physical abuse in pregnancy. *Obstet Gynecol* 1985;66:185–90.
2. Helton AS, Anderson E, McFarlane J. Battered and pregnant: a prevalence study with intervention measures. *Am J Public Health* 1987;77:1337–9.
3. Hedin LW, Grimstad H, Moller A, Schei B, Janson PO. Prevalence of physical and sexual assault before and during pregnancy among Swedish couples. *Acta Obstet Gynecol Scand* 1999;78:310–15.
4. McFarlane J, Parker B, Soeken K, Silva C, Reed S. Severity of abuse before and during pregnancy for African American, Hispanic, and Anglo women. *J Nurse Midwifery* 1999;44(2):139–44.
5. Webster J, Sweett S, Stolz TA. Domestic violence in pregnancy. A prevalence study. *Med J Aust* 1994;161:466–70.
6. McFarlane J, Parker B, Soeken K, Bullock L. Assessing for abuse during pregnancy: severity and frequency of injuries and associated entry into prenatal care. *JAMA* 1992;267:3176–8.
7. Hedin LW, Janson PO. Domestic violence during pregnancy. The prevalence of physical injuries, substance abuse, abortions and miscarriages. *Acta Obstet Gynecol Scand* 2000;79:625–30.
8. Spedding RL, McWilliams M, McNicholl BP, Dearden CH. Markers for domestic violence in women. *J Accid Emerg Med* 1999;16:400–2.
9. Hilberman E, Munson K. Sixty battered women. *Victimology* 1977-78;(2):460–70.
10. Dietz PM, Gazmararian JA, Goodwin MM, Johnson CH and Rochat RW. Delayed

entry into prenatal care: effect of physical violence. *Obstet Gynecol* 1997;90:221–4.

11. McFarlane J, Parker B, Soeken K. Abuse during pregnancy: association with maternal health and infant birth weight. *Nurs Res* 1996;45:37–42.

12. Greenberg EM, McFarlane J, Watson MG. Vaginal bleeding and abuse: assessing pregnant women in the emergency department. *MCN Am J Matern Child Nurs* 1997;22:182–6.

13. Mezey GC, Bewley S. *An Exploration of the Prevalence and Effects of Domestic Violence in Pregnancy.* London: Economic and Social Research Council; 2001. [www1.rhbnc.ac.uk/sociopolitical-science/vrp/Findings/rfmezey.pdf] Accessed 2 September 2003].

14. Satin AJ, Ramin SM, Paicurich J, Millman S, Wendel GD. The prevalence of sexual assault: a survey of 2404 puerperal women. *Am J Obstet Gynecol* 1992;167:973–5.

15. Berenson AB, Wiemann CM, Wilkinson GS, Jones WA, Anderson GD. Perinatal morbidity associated with violence experienced by pregnant women. *Am J Obstet Gynecol* 1994;170:1760–9.

16. Parker B, McFarlane J, Soeken K, Torres S and Campbell D. Physical and emotional abuse in pregnancy: a comparison of adult and teenage women. *Nurs Res* 1993;42:173–8.

17. Renker PR. Physical abuse, social support, self-care and pregnancy outcomes of older adolescents. *J Obstet Gynecol Neonatal Nurs* 1999;28:377–88.

18. Grimstad H, Shei B, Backe B, Jacobsen G. Interpersonal conflict and physical abuse in relation to pregnancy and infant birthweight. *J Womens Health Gend Based Med* 1999;8:847–53.

19. Campbell J, Torres S, Ryan J, King C, Campbell DW, Stallings RY *et al.* Physical and nonphysical partner abuse and other risk factors for low birth weight among full term and preterm: a multiethnic case-control study. *Am J Epidemiol* 1999;150:714–26.

20. McFarlane J, Parker B, Soeken K. Physical abuse, smoking and substance abuse during pregnancy: prevalence, interrelationships, and effects on birth weight. *J Obstet Gynecol Neonatal Nurs* 1996;25:313–20.

21. Fernandez FM, Krueger PM. Domestic violence: effect on pregnancy outcome. *J Am Osteopath Assoc* 1999;99:254–6.

22. Satin AJ, Hemsell DL, Stone IC, Theriot S, Wendel GD. Sexual assault in pregnancy. *Obstet Gynecol* 1991;77:710–14.

23. Shumway J, O'Campo P, Gielen A, Witter FR, Khouzami AN, Blakemore KJ. Preterm labor, placental abruption and premature rupture of membranes in relation to maternal violence or verbal abuse. *J Matern Fetal Med* 1999;8:76–80.

24. Jacoby M, Gorenflo D, Black E, Wunderlich C, Eyler AE. Rapid repeat pregnancy and experience of interpersonal violence among low-income adolescents. *Am J Prev Med* 1999;16:318–21.

25. Gazmararian JA, Saltzman LE, Johnson CH, Bruce FC, Marks JS, Zahniser SC. The relationship between pregnancy intendedness and physical violence in mothers of newborns. The PRAMS Working Group. *Obstet Gynecol* 1995;85:1031–8.

26. Glander SS, Moore ML, Michielutte R, Parsons LH. The prevalence of domestic violence among women seeking abortion. *Obstet Gynecol* 1998;91:1002–6.

27. Stewart DE. Incidence of postpartum abuse in women with a history of abuse during pregnancy. *Can Med Assoc J* 1994;1551:1602–4.

28. Gielen AC, O'Campo PJ, Faden RR, Kass NE, Xue X. Interpersonal conflict and physical violence during the childbearing year. *Soc Sci Med* 1994;39:781–7.

29. Martin SL. Physical abuse of women before, during, and after pregnancy. *JAMA* 2001;285:1581–4.

30. Holmes MM, Resnick HS, Kilpatrick DG, Best CL. Rape-related pregnancy: estimates and descriptive characteristics from a national sample of women. *Am J Obstet Gynecol* 1996;175:320–5.

31. Martinez AH, Villanueva LA, Torres C, Garcia LE. Sexual aggression in adolescents. Epidemiologic study. *Ginecol Obstet Mex* 1999;67:449–53.

32. Hammond HA, Redman JB, Caskey CT. In-utero paternity testing following alleged sexual assault. A comparison of DNA-based methods. *JAMA* 1995;273:1774–7.

33. Lewis G. Domestic violence. In: Lewis G, Drife J, editors. Why Mothers Die 1997–1999: Fifth Report of the Confidential Enquiries into Maternal Deaths in the United Kingdom. London: RCOG Press; 2001. p.241–51.

34. Kellerman AL, Mercy JA. Men, women and murder: gender-specific differences in rates of fatal violence and victimization. *J Trauma* 1992;33:1–5.

35. Parsons LH, Harper MA. Violent maternal deaths in North Carolina. *Obstet Gynecol* 1999;94:990–3.

36. National Collaborating Centre for Women's and Children's Health. *Antenatal Care: Routine Care for the Healthy Pregnant Woman*. London: RCOG Press; 2003.

37. Norton LB, Peipert JF, Zierler S, Lima B, Hume L. Battering in pregnancy: an assessment of two screening methods. *Obstet Gynecol* 1995;85:321–5.

38. Recognising Domestic Violence. The role of the health care professional. In: Department of Health. *Domestic Violence: A Resource Manual for Health Care Professionals*. London: Department of Health; March 2000. p. 19–41. [www.info.doh.gov.uk/doh/point.nsf/66b6f04bdca6defc0025693b0051ada0/d1e8b675f5 418c7b002566ff003ad69d/$FILE/domestic_violence.pdf] Accessed 2 September 2003.

39. Covington DL, Dalton VK, Diehl S, Wright BD, Piner MH. Improving detection of violence among pregnant adolescents. *J Adolesc Health* 1997;21:18–24.

40. Marchant S, Davidson LL, Garcia J, Parsons JE. Addressing domestic violence through maternity services: policy and practice. *Midwifery* 2000;17:164–70.

41. Parker B, McFarlane J, Soeken K, Silva C, Reel S. Testing an intervention to prevent further abuse to pregnant women. *Res Nurs Health* 1999;22:59–66.

42. McFarlane J, Wiist W. Preventing abuse to pregnant women: implementation of a 'mentor mother' advocacy model. *J Community Health Nurs* 1997;14:237–9.

43. Amaro H, Fried LE, Zuckerman B. Violence during pregnancy and substance abuse. *Am J Public Health* 1990; 80: 575–9.

44. O'Campo P, Gielen AC, Faden RR, Kass N. Verbal abuse and physical violence among a cohort of low-income pregnant women. *Womens Health Issues* 1994;4(1);29–37.

45. Muhajarine N, D'Arcy C. Physical abuse during pregnancy: prevalence and risk factors. *CMAJ* 1999;160:1007–1.

46. Johnson JK, Haider F, Ellis K, Hay DM, Lindow SW. The prevalence of domestic violence in pregnant women. *BJOG* 2003;110:272–5.

Chapter 14

The impact of domestic violence in gynaecology

Joseph Johnson and Stephen Lindow

Introduction

Domestic violence against women is a worldwide concern that has extensive health and social consequences. Despite its wide-reaching effects, domestic violence usually remains undetected or under-reported in healthcare and social settings. The impact of domestic violence on health is as important as smoking but, in contrast to smoking, it has been neglected by the medical profession.

As a public health issue, the cost implications in relation to domestic violence are incalculable in terms of both medical expense and time lost at work due to sickness and absenteeism. The total healthcare costs associated with battered women in the USA in 1980 was estimated at US$44.4 million.[1]

The current health service response is based on a medical model of health rather than a social model and, although there is a growing awareness about domestic violence, this has not been translated into effective action at the present time.

Prevalence

Domestic violence is so widespread that no social, demographic or economic strata are spared. The study patterns and data collection methods vary and these are reflected in the results from different prevalence studies. Definitions of domestic violence vary considerably, including differing personal relationships and differing degrees or types of violence (physical, sexual, emotional, etc.), which affects the results of prevalence studies. Although the magnitude of domestic violence is not known, a prevalence of between one in five and one in three is generally accepted as the likely number of women who have experienced violence.

The discrepancy between the likely numbers of women who are experiencing violence at home and the low detection rate is well known and documented. A review of medical records of patients attending general practices in the Hackney district of London showed a prevalence of 41% (425/1035) and 17% of these had experienced physical violence within the past year.[2]

With respect to the gynaecological practice in the UK, it is not precisely known how many conditions have their origin in domestic violence. However, given the known prevalence in general practice, it can be assumed that a gynaecologist must have significant numbers of patients with this background.

Presentation

The effects of domestic violence on women's health are varied and enormous. They are more likely to suffer from poor health, chronic pain, depression, addiction, and problem pregnancies, and to attempt suicide. Persistent gynaecological complaints, particularly abdominal pain and miscarriage, could be important presentations of abuse.[3]

A Norwegian study[4] reported an increased likelihood of gynaecological symptoms in abused women at the time of interview. Another general practice-based prevalence study indicated that women who had experienced domestic violence within the previous 12 months were more likely to have vaginal discharge, pelvic pain or genital pain.[5]

Anxiety, depression, sleeping difficulties, ill-defined illnesses, eating disorders, irritable bowel syndrome and headache are well documented in women who have been abused. They also make greater use of psychiatric, gynaecological and emergency services. Abuse may be the reason for failed clinic attendance, noncompliance with medication, depression and other unexplained physical and psychological signs and symptoms. Women who report domestic violence are disproportionately young, poor, unmarried, living with a male friend or family members other than their spouse. After controlling for other sociodemographic characteristics, intimate sexual violence is significantly related to poorer physical and mental health and increased problems with access to medical care.[6]

Sexual abuse has been linked to domestic violence. A study of domestic violence and sexual abuse in female physicians indicated that those reporting histories of domestic violence were significantly less likely to be single and significantly more likely to report suicide attempts, substance abuse, current or past smoking, severe daily stress at home, chronic fatigue syndrome, and their mothers were more likely to have experienced domestic violence.[7] Women with borderline personality disorders have been found to have suffered more intrafamilial physical and sexual abuse.[8]

Sexually abused women are at high risk of pelvic inflammatory disease (PID) and so the assessment for sexual abuse is an essential part of the clinical management of women with a diagnosis of PID. The combined prevalence of bacterial vaginosis and chlamydia was found to be significantly higher in abused women.[9] Sexually abused women are more likely to have lower incomes, earlier coitus, a history of sexually acquired infections, current abusive partner, new sex partners, anal sex and bleeding with sex.

Adolescents with a history of domestic violence were, in the past six months, 2.8 times more likely to have a sexually transmitted disease, 2.8 times more likely to have a non-monogamous male partner and half as likely to use condoms consistently; more likely to fear the perceived consequences of negotiating condom use; feared talking with their partner about pregnancy prevention; had a higher perceived risk of acquiring a sexually transmitted disease and perceived less control over their sexuality.[10]

The presentation may also be subtle; most individuals with chronic fatigue syndrome report a past history of interpersonal abuse. Physical and sexual abuse may lead to derangement of neuroendocrine functions, thereby affecting ovarian function and potentially leading to altered age at perimenopausal transition.[11]

The family of origin of the wife may be an important predisposition for problem in adult life. A detailed review of risk markers in husband-to-wife violence found that only witnessing violence in the wife's family of origin as a child or adolescent was consistently associated with being subsequently victimised by violence.[12] Other studies show that early and repeated sexual abuse in the family of origin may be associated with later domestic violence.[13]

Despite the numerous assumptions described above, most demographic features are not useful aids in identifying individual woman experiencing domestic violence, as they are not specific. Presence of certain features in the woman's past history raises the likelihood of her experiencing domestic violence.

Physician's awareness

As stated, the risk factors for domestic violence are sensitive but not specific enough to be clinically useful in identifying women who are experiencing domestic violence. Thus, there is a failure of recognition of domestic violence on the part of health workers and this may be compounded by lack of awareness.

It is possible that a physician may not have the time to devote to the problem and may also lack the knowledge and skills to cope adequately. Legal implications may prevent a physician becoming involved and the sum of the associated problems may lead to the conclusion that it is not a good use of time.

From the perspective of the woman, fear of retaliation from the abusive partner and limitations of the care system may be the factors that inhibit a woman from voluntarily disclosing domestic violence. She may also believe that clinicians lack time and interest in discussing abuse and may have concerns about confidentiality. Police and legal involvement may also concern some women and prevent disclosure.

Studies show that primary care physicians are less likely to screen for domestic violence than gynaecologists.[14] Thirty percent of physicians hold a victim-blame attitude and 70% do not believe that they have the resources available to them to assist victims.[15]

In a survey in the USA, the majority of obstetric and gynaecological resident programme directors revealed that they had integrated or intended to integrate an American College of Obstetricians and Gynecologists learning module on domestic violence into their residents' and medical students' formal curricula.[16]

Treatment implications

The United Nations General Assembly passed a declaration on the Elimination of Violence against Women in 1993, describing such violence as an historical manifestation of the unequal power relationship between men and women. South Africa's first democratic government passed a domestic violence Act into law in 1998 as a part of local and international commitment to protecting the human rights of women. In the UK, a national Agenda for Action was drawn up following the United Nations Fourth Assembly Congress in 1993.

Effective detection and intervention for domestic violence has always been a problem in any part of the world and the biggest hurdle may be the constitution of the healthcare system, particularly the lack of integration between the medical and social service networks. Although the signs of domestic violence are apparent, medical professionals generally feel less confident and not appropriately supported to deal with these complex social problems and many times fail to intervene effectively. Women's general fear of disclosure and denial also contribute to the physician's reluctance to pursue the matter.

The barriers within the healthcare sector have to be dealt with on three different levels:

- the structural level, in order to diminish male power in society
- the organisational level, in order to initiate screening and allow staff time to deal with the victims
- an individual level, to empower women to disclose abuse.[17]

In less obvious situations, the attention is diverted to the secondary health problems associated with domestic violence, both physical and psychological, while the primary underlying factors are overlooked. Effective management of domestic violence should not be restricted to mere treatment of the presenting physical symptoms but should involve a wider integration of the clinician's efforts with appropriate recognition of the impact of social factors.

The role of the gynaecologist

The gynaecologist has a definite role to play. One should exercise the utmost caution and show a fair degree of sensitivity. Although the presence of abuse may be obvious, a woman will commonly deny it. Lack of privacy and confidentiality may contribute to this denial of domestic violence.

The presence of a family member or a dominant partner may inhibit communication about past gynaecological or obstetric history, marital or sexual problems or domestic violence.[18] The presence of a chaperone may intrude in a confidential doctor–patient relationship and may reduce a doctor's acuity in detecting nonverbal signs of distress from the patient.[18]

A good doctor acknowledges the woman's feelings and is alert to the nonverbal clues. Doctors can offer help to a woman who has disclosed domestic violence in three main ways:

- respect and validation
- assessment of immediate physical problems and further actions
- information about where to find help.

If domestic violence is apparent, the injuries should be assessed and recorded; further danger should be evaluated. A safety plan should ideally be discussed with the woman and emergency contact numbers should be given.

Routine screening

In one survey, when asked, women generally welcomed the introduction of routine questioning about domestic violence in clinical settings.[19] A study from Queensland, Australia, showed that 98% of women believed it was a good idea to screen for domestic violence.[20] Barriers for 'screening' for domestic violence include a lack of information and attitude problems. Interdisciplinary methods of formal education, in-service training and continuing education are encouraged to augment or initiate universal screening.[21]

Questions about domestic violence should be included in clinical consultations. Areas that should be emphasised during a domestic violence training programme include appropriate history, necessary physical examination, documenting the injuries and reporting the issues to the concerned authority.

A system model approach improved the domestic violence service in a managed care setting within one year and affected clinicians' behaviour as well as health plan members' experiences.[22] This successful implementation made it possible to evaluate research questions about the impact of a health-care intervention for victims of domestic violence in a managed healthcare setting.

Training

Staff are reluctant to ask sensitive questions about domestic violence. They may be worried that this may appear rude and may feel that they do not have the training to deal with a positive response. Healthcare professionals do not routinely receive appropriate training before and after qualification and, as a result, may provide inadequate care to women who have experienced domestic violence. A significant increase was seen in the willingness of healthcare professionals to assess and intervene with battered pregnant women after an educational programme.[23] Since training does appear to be associated with better screening, educational tools should be improved to specifically address these barriers.

Training programmes are designed to improve the awareness and understanding of domestic violence, to provide information about agencies that provide support for women, to consider attitudes to domestic violence and to acquire tools to implement protocols effectively and systematically in the work setting.[24] Based upon published reports, it appears that few rigorously designed evaluations have been conducted of training programmes for health providers in the detection and treatment of women affected by domestic violence.[25]

Management controversies

National priorities

Domestic violence should be recognised at a national level as an issue for health services and those responsible for the training of healthcare professionals. This goal revision requires education on the dynamics of domestic violence, confrontation of personal issues and formation of common partnerships. Implications include the development of curricula and protocols to create a united front against domestic violence within the healthcare, social support and law enforcement communities.

Treatment strategies

Screening for any condition is only appropriate if there is an acceptable treatment for it. Once domestic violence is identified, appropriately responding to the woman's needs presents other problems. Although guidelines (DOH,[26] ACOG[27]) about domestic violence are in place, most physicians do not provide all the services recommended for women who have been abused. Guidelines and protocols should be tested in an intervention trial to determine whether their use would lead to increased screening and improved management of abuse.

If domestic violence is found, is it possible to correct this behaviour in the relationship? Men who completed treatment in a programme for spouse abuse showed more commitment, better working capacities and a higher level of agreement with their therapists.[28] However, the successful men were better educated and had better economic conditions.

Multidisciplinary approach

A strategic approach should be adopted as the basis for improving the health service's response to the issue of domestic violence.[24] This approach is based on a policy framework to standardise good practice across different services. The service is delivered through community-based multidisciplinary clinics and is both appropriate and sensitive to the needs of women who are experiencing domestic violence.

Audit in different departments may help to analyse the methods for improved detection and response to women who are experiencing domestic violence and also to evaluate Home Office recommendations for introducing protocols on domestic violence in conjunction with staff training within the health service.

Blame culture

Little work has been done on the origins of domestic violence. Some authors in the late 1970s and early 1980s tried to view domestic violence in terms of 'individual pathology',[29,30] with emphasis on provoking the masochistic and violence-seeking nature of those women involved.[31] Some observational studies suggested that most women who experience violence in their relations came from a violent background and had seen or experienced this behaviour from an early age. Women were seen as addicted to violence and often provoking it and seeking out such encounters.

There is no solid evidence for the role 'individual pathology'. The community prevalence study by Andrews and Brown,[32] who adopted a biographical approach, emphasised the lack of evidence to support the idea that women who experience marital violence were 'addicted' to it. Moreover, in terms of wider social influence, this negative attitude is inappropriate and detracts interest away from the pertinent issues.

Is it the gynaecologist's job?

Many studies have shown that doctors do not ask about domestic violence routinely. Lack of time and training are the principal barriers. Some cast doubt on the appropriateness of the gynaecologist as the health worker who should screen and intervene on the subject of domestic violence. Many physicians have stated that it was not their place to intrude into sensitive personal areas. With the implementation of clinical governance and the increasing expectations of patients, doctors find themselves with heightened responsibility and a struggle to find enough time to deal with these problems. Better methods to convince gynaecologists of the relevance of abuse to their practices and to help them incorporate the management of abuse into their already busy schedules need to be developed.

One approach could be to designate a nurse practitioner or a health worker as resource person for violence in a particular setting, who would become familiar with the management of victims, community resources and local counsellors who are experienced in abuse.[33]

Frequent admissions may be more an indicator of a woman's distress or fear than of a specific medical concern. Guidelines and pathways should be set for screening women who attend with recurrent gynaecological symptoms of abdominal discomfort, pelvic pain, vaginal discharge and genitourinary infections and arrangements should be made for appropriate referral to a domestic violence coordinator.

Conclusion

There are moral, financial and legal imperatives for the detection of survivors of domestic violence when they attend with recurrent and nonspecific gynaecological symptoms.

Early research into routine screening for domestic violence shows a significant increase in the willingness of healthcare professionals to assess and assist battered women. Doctors can offer help to a woman who has disclosed domestic violence by giving her respect and validation, by assessing her immediate physical problems and giving her information about where to get help.[33]

Guidelines and protocols for the care of women experiencing domestic violence have been used in healthcare settings in the USA from the late 1970s. A multidisciplinary approach may be necessary, with referral to appropriate agencies for women traumatised by sexual abuse or domestic violence and for those requiring psychosexual counselling. A new collaboration between epidemiologists, policy makers, researchers, practitioners and health professionals could lead to more successful ways of identifying abuse.

References

1.   Inter-university Consortium for Political and Social Research. *The National Crime Survey in the USA*. Ann Arbor, MI: ICPSR; 1981.
2.   Richardson J, Coid J, Petruckevitch A, Chung WS, Moorey S. Identifying domestic violence: cross sectional study in primary care. *BMJ* 2002;324:274.
3.   Stark E, Flitcraft. A. *Women at Risk*. London: Sage; 1996.
4.   Schie B, Bakketeig LS. Gynaecological impact of sexual and physical abuse by spouse. A study of a random sample of Norwegian women. *BJOG* 1989;96:1379–83.
5.   McCauley J, Kern DE, Kolodner K, Dill L, Schroeder AF, DeChant HK, *et al.* The "battering syndrome": prevalence and clinical characteristics of domestic violence in primary care internal medicine practices. *Ann Intern Med* 1995;123:737–46.
6.   Plichta S. Prevalence of violence and its implications for women's health. *Womens Health Issues* 2001;11(3):244–58.
7.   Doyle JP, Frank E, Saltzman LE, McMohan PM, Fielding BD. Domestic violence and sexual abuse in women physicians: associated medical, psychiatric, and professional difficulties. *J Womens Health Gend Based Med* 1999;8:955–65.

8.   Laporte L, Guttman H. Abusive relationship in families of women with borderline personality disorder, anorexia nervosa and a control group. *J Nerv Ment Dis* 2001;189:522–31.

9.   King EA, Britt R, McFarlane JM, Hawkins C. Bacterial vaginosis and chlamydia trachomatis among pregnant abused and non-abused Hispanic women. *J Obstet Gynecol Neonatal Nurs* 2000;29:606–12.

10.   Wingood GM, DiClemente RJ, McCree DH, Harrington K. Dating violence and the sexual health of black adolescent females. *Paediatrics* 2001;107:E72.

11.   Allsworth JE, Zierler S, Krieger N, Harlow BL. Ovarian function in late reproductive years in relation to lifetime experience of abuse. *Epidemiology* 2001;12:676–81.

12.   Hotaling GT, Sugarman D. An analysis of risk markers in husband to wife violence: the current state of knowledge. *Violence Vict* 1986;1:101–24.

13.   Plitcha. Effects of women abuse on health care utilisation and health status: a literature review. *Womens Health Issues* 1992;2:154–63.

14.   Rodriguez MA, Bauer HM, McLoughlin E, Grumbach K. Screening and intervention for intimate partner abuse: practise and attitudes of primary care physicians. *JAMA* 1999;282:468–74.

15.   Garimella R, Plitchta SB, Houseman C, Garzon L. Physician's belief about victims of spouse abuse and the physician's role. *J Womens Health Gend Based Med* 2000;9:405–11.

16.   Chez RA, Horan DL. Response of obstetrics and gynaecology program directors on domestic violence lecture module. *Am J Obstet Gynecol* 1999;180:496–8.

17.   Ronnberg AK, Hammarstrom A. Barriers within the health care system to dealing with sexualised violence: a literature review. *Scand J Public Health* 2000;28:222–9.

18.   Crowley P. Sensitive vaginal examination. *Violence Against Women*. London: RCOG Press; 1997. p. 262–79.

19.   Bradley F, Smith M, Long J, O'Dowd T. Reported frequency of domestic violence: cross sectional survey on women attending general practice. *BMJ* 2002;324:271.

20.   Webster J, Stratigos SM, Grimes KM. Women's responses to screening for domestic violence in a secondary care setting. *Midwifery* 2001;17:289–94.

21.   Davis RE, Harsh KE. Confronting barriers to universal screening for domestic violence. *J Prof Nurs* 2001;17:313–20.

22.   McCaw B, Berman WH, Syme SL, Hunkeler EF. Beyond screening for domestic violence: a system model approach in a managed care setting. *Am J Prev Med* 2001;21:170–6.

23.   Helton A, McFarlane J. Prevention of battering during pregnancy: focus on behavioural change. *Public Health Nurs* 1987;4:166–74.

24.   Hepburn M, McCartney S. Domestic Violence and reproductive health care in Glasgow. *Violence Against Women*. London: RCOG Press; 1997. p. 233–44.

25.   Davidson LL, Grisso JA, Garcia J, King VJ. Training programmes for healthcare professionals in domestic violence. *J Womens Health Gend Based Med* 2001;10:953–69.

26.   Department of Health. *Domestic Violence: A Resource Manual for Health Professionals*. London: DoH; 2000 [www.doh.gov.uk/domestic.htm].

27.   ACOG guidelines on domestic violence.

28.   Rondeau G, Brodeur N, Brochu S, Lemire G. Dropout and completion of treatment among spouse abusers. *Violence Vict* 2001;16:127–43.

29.   Freeman MD. The phenomenon of marital violence and the legal and social response in England. In: Freeman MD. *Family Violence*. Toronto: Butterworth; 1979.

30.   Pizzey E, Shapiro J. *Prone to Violence*. London: Hamlyn; 1982.

31.   Gayford JJ. Wife battering: a preliminary survey. *BMJ* 1979;i:194–7.

32.   Andrew B, Brown G W. Marital violence in the community. A biographical approach. *Br J Psychiatr* 1988;153:305–12.

33.   Richardson J, Feder G. How can we help? The role of general practice. *Violence Against Women*. London: RCOG Press; 1997. p. 157–67.

Chapter 15

The doctor's role

Lindsey Stevens

Introduction

The essence of an abusive relationship is that one partner seeks to control the other. Physical control is exerted by assault, including sexual assault, the use of weapons and restraint[1,2] and by the enrolment of the victim in substance abuse. Emotional control is exerted by threatening suicide, abandonment and violence to the victim or children; by isolating the victim from friends and family; by repeated denigration; by controlling money and the freedom to move (e.g. by holding a passport or threatening exposure of illegal immigrant status);[3] and by manipulating the victim's need for admiration and affection by professions of love and commitment, gifts and attention to the children.[4] This combination of physical and emotional coercion creates feelings of fear, entrapment[5] and disempowerment in the victim,[6] which express themselves through a variety of stress-related medical and physical problems and difficulty in accessing help. The gratifying aspects of the relationship create confusion and ambivalence in the victim's evaluation of their situation.[7,8,9] The alternation between abuse and apparent affection has been characterised as the 'cycle of violence'.[4] The latter consists of a tension building phase, the explosion of violence and then a phase of apology and rapprochement.

Presentation

There is ample evidence, both in the UK and abroad, that domestic violence poses considerable demands on the National Health Service, costing the nation many millions every year.[10] The impact of domestic violence on obstetrics and gynaecology has been detailed in the preceding chapters. The effects on other groups of patients are widespread and significant,[11] with victims of abuse presenting not just with trauma but being highly represented within the symptom groups that make up the 'unpopular patient',[12] such as those with pain that does not respond to surgical or medical intervention[13] and those with recurrent deliberate self-harm.[14] Box

15.1 lists some of the more common nontraumatic presentations in general medicine and surgery.

Box 15.1

Symptoms commonly experienced by victims of abuse who present to general medical or surgical practice[13,15–22]

- Gastro-oesophageal reflux
- Irritable bowel syndrome
- Chest pain
- Syncope
- Dysuria
- Breast pain
- Chronic headache
- Hyperventilation
- Unexplained body pain or somatisation
- Backache
- Chronic pain
- Delayed recovery from surgery
- Unsuccessful symptom relief
- Multiple operations

Gastrointestinal symptoms are particularly common. Drossman *et al.*[18,23] found that women with irritable bowel syndrome who had a history of abuse exhibited greater symptom reporting and health use and that abuse victims were 92% of women who presented with gastro-oesophageal reflux and 82% of women with irritable bowel syndrome.

The psychological impact of domestic violence is marked,[24] leading to eating and sleeping disorders, depression,[25] anxiety,[26] post-traumatic stress symptoms,[27] panic attacks[28] and parasuicide or suicide.[29–31] A history of any of these disorders or of the taking of antidepressant medication[32] is a pointer. Studies have revealed that 68% of psychiatric outpatients[33] and 81% of inpatients had a history of abuse.[34] Up to 45% of female alcoholics and 50% of female drug abusers are also battered women[35] and between 7%[24]and 16%[5] of women in violent relationships have been found to abuse drugs or alcohol.

Deliberate self-harm is thought to be triggered by a situation that is perceived to have three components: defeat, no escape and no rescue.[36] Being trapped in a violent home certainly fulfils these criteria. In this context, the act of self harm acts "as a cry for help, as a means to exercise some control in their lives, as a punishment for being such a guilty person, and as an inwardly directed expression of anger".[37] Sexual abuse appears to be a major trigger factor.[38]

Where the woman has sought help for an injury, the mechanism of injury offered may be inconsistent with the injury. Injury is much more likely to be to the head (particularly face), neck, chest (especially breasts), and abdomen (especially genitalia), and far less likely to involve a lower limb, than injury to a woman who has not been abused.[39,40] Punching, pushing, slapping and assault with an object were common mechanisms of injury,[39] with contusions and internal injury being heavily associated with abuse, and sprains and strains with nonabuse.[41] The evidence on upper-limb injuries and fractures is mixed, with some studies finding upper limb injury to be a marker of abuse and limb fractures more common[42] and some not.[41] Spiral or healing fractures should raise suspicion, as should burns, bites and scalds. Injuries are likely to be multiple, of differing ages, and may be symmetrical.

Chronic illnesses such as asthma, ischaemic heart disease, diabetes and hypertension may be worsened by the stress of an abusive relationship.[43]

Prevalence studies conducted in general emergency departments record 1.2–11.7% of attendances to be due to the effects of domestic violence on the day and 14.0–54.2% of patients to have been victims of domestic violence at some time.[44-54] The British Crime Survey of 1996 found that 4.2% of those they interviewed had experienced domestic violence within the preceding year and that 26% of women and 17% of men had experienced it at some time; 47% of female homicide victims were killed by their partner or ex-partner and 43% of all violent crime experienced by women was domestic. In total the survey estimated that there were 6.6 million incidents of domestic violence in 1995.[55]

A woman's risk of being injured by a partner or ex-partner has been estimated at 22%, with 9% being severely injured.[56] In a study of female assault victims, 41% had been assaulted by their partner, ex-partner or another family member.[53] Domestic violence is the most common cause of nonfatal injury in the USA.[57] A study in primary care found a lifetime prevalence of 41% among women.[58]

A woman currently suffering domestic violence can be of any age but is likely to be aged between 16 and 39 years[49,55] and single (particularly separated or divorced).[55] Social vulnerability, e.g. young children in the home, financial difficulties, homelessness, disability, illegal immigrant status and limited English are also risk factors.[1,49,55,59] Recurrent attendances at primary care or emergency facilities,[60] particularly for injury, should arouse concern as should the taking of multiple medications. One study found that 80% of women who attended the emergency department more than three times with injury were victims of domestic assault.[35] Having said this, abuse occurs to women of all classes, ages and races and should always be considered. Risk factors are cumulative: a teenager who is pregnant is at higher risk than an older woman of abuse and an abused, pregnant teenager is much more likely to turn to substance abuse than one who is not.[61]

The victim is likely to be passive, vague, evasive, guarded, embarrassed and apologetic.[4] She may be over-vehement when denying abuse.

Delayed presentation after the violent incident is the rule rather than the exception. Campbell *et al.*'s study[60] of the use of emergency departments by shelter residents revealed that, while 93% suffered chronic mental or physical health problems, 63% had not attended an accident and emergency department immediately subsequent to an attack. This was confirmed by another study, which found that 68% of women suffering domestic violence did not seek help at the time of their injuries.[45] Attendance tends to be out-of-hours.[41]

Interviewing the woman

It is vital to interview the woman on her own; indeed, reluctance to allow this by her partner is itself an indicator.[62] Excluding the partner may be difficult and calls for some creative thinking by the physician. A departmental policy of always initially assessing a patient without accompanying persons is helpful; the companion may be brought in after the examination for further discussion. The partner may not, however, accept such a policy, in which case strategies such as moving the patient to an area such as X-ray, ultrasound or a treatment room may allow exclusion of the partner under the guise of 'health and safety'. Asking the partner to check registration details at the reception desk or involving him in discussion with another health professional (e.g. on whether he has any worries about his partner's condition which he would like to discuss) may create an opportunity for private discussion with the woman. Should none of these ruses work and the physician is concerned, then admission to a day unit or observation facility, or even warding, may be the only way of buying space and time to talk to the patient properly. The woman who speaks poor English is an exception to the rule of interviewing alone. It is advisable to use a hospital translator or ethnic link worker, rather than an accompanying friend or relative, as the woman may feel inhibited in discussing her situation in front of people linked to her home life.

Most victims of domestic violence find it difficult to discuss their problems.[63,64] The reasons include feelings of humiliation, helplessness and self-blame, lowered self-esteem, denial (rationalisation of the violence), concern for others such as the children, fear of the perpetrator, uncertainty about the future and a lack of resources. The victim may have little knowledge of the support available or negative experiences of seeking help from the police or health services in the past.

The evidence is that victims are unlikely to reveal their experience without active prompting. Studies of disclosure find that only around 25% of victims self-report their abuse.[65] However, if women are asked direct questions about domestic violence, they are much more likely to disclose,[66] especially if asked repeatedly.[67] The evidence is that such questioning is welcome. One study found that 96% of patients attending an emergency department[68] accepted being asked about their experience of domestic violence. This was borne out by a study that found only 5.6%[54] of woman who were uncomfortable or very uncomfortable when asked such questions. Women themselves often list medical services as their main or preferred source of help.[69-71]

The woman should be asked direct questions gently and reassured that domestic violence is common, that asking about it is routine and that the health service is an appropriate place to come for help. An example of such questioning would be, in response to a pregnant patient presenting with an abdominal trauma that she said was caused by slipping in the kitchen, "I know that you have told me that your injury was caused by a fall but I must tell you that I see this kind of injury much more commonly after an assault than a fall. Most of these assaults happen in the home, and pregnancy is a particularly common time for them to happen. Is this what has happened to you?".

The physician must then reassure their patient that anything they discuss will not be revealed to the partner and is in confidence. Whether this confidentiality is in fact absolute is a dilemma that is discussed later in this chapter. However, all care must be taken to prevent the partner finding out that any such discussions have taken place. The practice of patient-held records in obstetric care represents a risk and care must be taken what is entered in the case-notes.

The physician must also bear in mind the forensic significance of their examination and notes, whether or not the victim intends to take action against the perpetrator at that time. Records must include the time, date and place of assault and any witnesses to it; the size, pattern, age, description and location of injury, evidence of non-bodily abuse, such as torn clothes, destruction of the victim's possessions, violence to pets and verbal abuse. Photographs are helpful and should be taken within the guidelines summarised in Box 15.2.

Forensic evidence, such as torn clothing, pieces of glass or weapons must be preserved. Ideally, they should be passed directly to the police. If this is not possible, the items should be placed in a sealed bag that is dated, timed and signed by the person putting the evidence in the bag. Every time the evidence is passed to another person, the handover must be recorded on the bag, with the handover dated, timed and signed by both the donor and the recipient. If at any time this 'chain of evidence' is broken the evidence may not be admissible in court. See Chapters 6–8.

The physician should also record the woman's explanation of her injuries (commencing this record with, 'patient states'), their own opinion of the cause of injury if the injury seems inconsistent with the patient's explanation and known characteristics of the abuser, such as a criminal or psychiatric history and alcohol or drug abuse.

Box 15.2

Protocol for the taking of photographs

- Explain to the woman that:
    - ☐ the photographs will be useful evidence in any present or future legal action
    - ☐ they will form part of the medical record and will only be released with the woman's permission.
- Obtain written consent from the woman, including the phrase "These photographs will only be released if and when the undersigned gives written permission to release the medical records".
- Take good-quality, well-lit photos, both from a distance so that the victim is identifiable and from close-up to detail the injuries.
- The photographer should sign and date the back of each photo.
- Place the photographs in a sealed envelope attached securely to the patient's records. Mark the envelope with the date and the notation "Photographs of patient's injury".
- Advise the woman to have further photographs taken in two or three days' time when bruising will be more evident (the police can arrange to do this, or the woman may be offered medical photography if she is unwilling to involve the police).

Advising the woman

The thrust of medical training is to identify a problem and then intervene to solve or at least control it.[72] An authoritarian approach of this sort merely compounds the disempowerment that accompanies abuse. Advice must be tailored to the woman's preparedness to accept and use it and must take into account the stage of the abusive relationship. Behaviour change occurs in stages:

- an initial difficulty in recognising a problem (precontemplation)
- then acknowledgement of the problem without being able to construct a solution (contemplation)
- then gathering of information and getting ready to confront the problem (preparation)
- then implementing the plan (action)
- and finally trying to sustain the change (maintenance).

Intervention tailored for one stage when the woman is at another will fail or even alienate her.[73] The physician's goal must be the empowerment of the woman to improve her safety, health and happiness[70,74–76] and this means that the physician must move at the woman's pace.

The assumption that the only good result is that the woman leaves the abusive relationship may be a misassumption for some women. There is evidence that the highest risk of serious injury or death is at the time of, or shortly after, leaving the abuser.[1,22,77] The substantial investment that the woman has made in her relationship, particularly when she has children, should not be discounted.[78] The systematic isolation perpetrated by abusers often means that women have no financial independence[5] and have been prevented from acquiring the skills that would make them independent. Constant denigration makes a woman feel that she would not be able to find work or another partner if she left.[79]

The physician should express concern and explore the woman's perception of her situation, particularly the risk that the perpetrator will seriously injure or kill her, any escalation in the frequency or level of violence, the presence of weapons in the home, any threat of or actual abuse of the children and any threatening behaviour towards family, friends or neighbours.[34,74] The evidence is that the cycle of violence[4] gets briefer in duration and the violence more severe each time. The effect of violence on the woman's general mental and physical health should also be discussed.

During these discussions the physician must remain non-judgemental. The most common result of an interview with a victim of domestic violence is that they return to the abuser, even if they initially separate. The decision to leave normally accompanies a landmark, such as children reaching school age or becoming involved in the violence.[1] Davies *et al.*[1] found that the interval between deciding to leave and permanent separation averaged eight years, with women leaving and returning, on average, five times. Many victims have had bad experiences of social services or the police in the past, many are afraid that they will be reported to the child protection team or that they may have to put their children into care if, by leaving their partner, they make themselves and their children homeless. Reporting violence to the police can increase the risk of future victimisation, even if the perpetrator is arrested.[80] Seeking help for mental health problems resulting from abuse may work against the woman in custody proceedings and mental illness or substance abuse can militate against a woman finding a place in a refuge.[78,81] Finally, the physician who has wholeheartedly condemned the abuser is unlikely to be the physician the woman consults when she is abused again.

In place of telling the woman what to do, the physician should explore with her what support she has sought before, whether she has separated from or attempted to separate from her partner in the past, what happened when she did and what choices and resources she believes she has available to her. Information on other options should be offered. These options include redress under both civil and criminal law.

Part IV of the Family Law Act 1996 sets out a range of measures available to the family courts under the civil law regarding domestic violence. Sections 33–41 set out the factors that are taken into account in occupation orders. These orders decide who should remain in the family home and who may be asked to leave. The risk of harm to the applicant is one of the factors considered. Section 42 empowers the court to grant a nonmolestation order. Section 47 adds a power of arrest to these orders.

Under criminal law, an assault between partners or within the home is now treated on the same basis as an assault between strangers. The perpetrator can be charged with the offences of common assault, grievous bodily harm, and so forth, and is subject to sentencing on the basis of the severity of the injury. Most police stations now have a domestic violence unit or domestic violence officers. These services have been shown to greatly improve the response of the police to victims.[82] The units often have a dedicated telephone line and should be the first point of contact for victims with the police.

Family law is a specialist area of legal work and victims may have difficulty contacting a lawyer in this field, particularly if they need a free initial consultation. Sources of contacts are police domestic violence units and the local domestic violence forum. The Law Society keeps lists of specialist lawyers in each area of legal work. The Citizen's Advice Bureau offers free legal advice.

As well as discussing the legal option of removal of the perpetrator from the home, the physician should discuss the woman's options if they leave themselves. Family or friends may be one option, but part of the process of abuse is to isolate the abused from their social supports[63] and many women have become distanced from their family and friends or may be frightened of putting them at risk from the perpetrator. The physician should be aware of other options locally such as refuges run by Women's Aid and other organisations, emergency housing through the social services, or, *in extremis*, a safe house provided through the police.

If the woman is returning to her partner, the physician should focus on crisis safety planning.[1,59,60,65,75] The woman should be provided with telephone numbers for sources of support. Most local domestic violence groups now produce a credit-card-sized list of key local agency numbers such as the police domestic violence unit and the local branch of Women's Aid. The woman should also be advised to keep important documents, such as her passport and rent book, hidden. Finally, if the woman is intending to leave at some stage, it is helpful if the physician talks through an exit strategy. Box 15.3 suggests some components of this.

If it is safe to do so, the woman should be encouraged to talk over her plans with her children so that they are prepared. She should leave when her partner is absent, if possible, but plans should be made that reflect the reality that she and the children might have to leave in haste at any time of the day or night.

The physician should gain the woman's agreement to her GP being informed of her situation. As well as the police, Women's Aid, social services and legal help, referral can usefully be made to Rape Crisis, Victim Support, family planning services and local drug and alcohol abuse teams.

Dilemmas

A block to discussing domestic violence is the lack of a shared agenda for that discussion, due to the variety of definitions of the term. The definition

Box 15.3

Components of an exit plan

- Where could you go to quickly use a telephone – friend, neighbour, family?
- Establish a code with family or friends, e.g. a particular phrase used during a telephone-call which is ostensibly about something else, to indicate you need help and agree in advance what help your contact will provide e.g. police, coming round, collecting children from school, etc.
- Ask a neighbour to call the police if they hear violence begin.
- Put together a bag containing the following; leave it outside the home with someone you trust and you can access in a hurry:
  - ☐ a list of the support numbers given plus other essential numbers – children's school, friend, etc.
  - ☐ an extra set of house, car and other essential keys
  - ☐ a set of clothes for yourself and for the children
  - ☐ any medications that you or the children need
  - ☐ essential legal and financial papers, e.g. birth certificates, passport, driving licence, benefit books, rent book, bank cards and account numbers
  - ☐ enough money to get you through at least a couple of days
  - ☐ small possessions of particular financial or sentimental value
  - ☐ favourite toys for the children.

of domestic violence used by the Department of Health in drawing up its generic guidelines for health workers is "physical, sexual or emotional abuse of a person by another with whom they have, or have had, an intimate relationship".[83] To simplify discussion and comparative data, it is suggested that this definition be used as the standard one among health workers in this country.

Screening

The first dilemma facing the clinician is whether to attempt to identify victims of domestic violence at all. Much of the controversy in this area[84,85] is due to ambiguity in the use of the word 'screening'. Several writers have used it in the sense of routinely asking patients about their home circumstances rather than screening in the strict public health sense applied to, for instance, cervical cancer screening. Several incidence or prevalence studies have described the use of 'screening' tools but the studies themselves do not fulfil the criteria of the UK National Screening Committee.[86] In fact, it could be argued that no studies fulfil these criteria in that an "effective treatment or intervention for the problem" is not yet defined. Support for the lack of utility of 'screening' is based partly on health professionals' reluctance to screen.[54]

So, wherein lies the reluctance of health professionals to tackle this issue? The fear of offending the patient, inadequate training, time constraints and a feeling of being unable to treat the problem have been found to be leading reasons why physicians do not discuss domestic violence with their patients.[54,68,87–91]

In addition, for some staff, discussing domestic violence with a woman may create personal distress. Given the prevalence of domestic violence in society, it is inevitable that a sizeable proportion of health professionals will have experienced violence within their own relationships at some stage. Estimates of the frequency of such experience lie between 10% and 38%.[92,93] Support for staff must be available before a general policy of enquiring about violence in the home is pursued.[94]

Tentativeness about asking women for details of their private lives is probably less significant a factor than anxiety about identifying a need which the professional does not know how to meet.[74,94] Few undergraduate training courses include the subject of domestic violence and it is missing from the postgraduate training curricula of many key specialties.[64,95] Even brief training courses have been shown to significantly increase staff members' knowledge base and willingness to explore domestic violence issues with patients.[96]

The heavy and unpredictable workloads of gynaecological, obstetric, emergency departments and primary care, coupled with the imposition of government throughput targets, which are grounded in quantity not quality concepts (six minutes per patient in primary care, all emergency department patients to have completed assessment, treatment and discharge or warding within four hours, with an average throughput of 75 minutes[97]), militate against staff in these areas developing new practices. Asking about domestic violence, when it receives a negative response, adding an esteem building statement and giving a leaflet about domestic violence takes less than 30 seconds. However, changing practice is perceived as increasing workload and stress and requiring time and commitment.[54] For many staff in an overstretched service, another protocol feels like a last straw. There may also be competition between practices that are introduced contemporaneously and staff feel defeated by being pulled in different directions and by the plethora of expectations of their performance. Staff also have legitimate concerns about the potential effects of delays for other patients if a large amount of time is spent with one patient, and may also have concerns about the aggression that may be directed towards them by those delayed patients. However, the greatest block to the involvement of any kind of professional in this field is probably the perceived lack of effective intervention.

In challenging violence in the home, the health professional is occupied in primary, secondary and tertiary prevention. Primary prevention lies in the message given to the wider community that violence between partners is noticed and is not to be tolerated. It is not many decades since the same message was sent out about child abuse and no-one would now say that health professionals have no obligation to identify children at risk and intervene immediately and vigorously.

The success of secondary or tertiary prevention is hard to quantify due to the lack of defined outcome measures. There is much work to do in this area before there can be any meaningful discussion of the efficacy of intervention. There is a great deal of evidence that relatively simple enquiry increases the identification of victims of domestic violence[98] but little evaluation of intervention methods or outcomes. Most victims of domestic violence continue to live with their partners and many episodes of violence occur before help is sought. An outcome of cessation of violence after a single intervention is not therefore realistic. One population measure might be the average number of episodes of violence before the victim is identified or seeks help. A decrease would represent a major improvement, although the experience of the individual health professional would still be that their patients usually return to their abusers. Measures of the health of individual women could include mental health status, symptom reporting in conditions such as irritable bowel syndrome and the frequency and severity of abusive incidents. The rare systematic study of outcome indicates intervention is advantageous.[99]

Whatever the debate, the public expects health professionals to offer help. In one study, 75% of patients attending a general practice expected the doctor to enquire about violence in the home. In contrast, only 33% of the doctors interviewed in the general practice thought they should actively enquire and only 7% actually had.[87] The studies mentioned above reveal that almost all patients attending emergency departments think that healthcare staff should enquire about domestic violence.[54,68] This expectation has been backed by professional bodies. The Department of Health,[1] the Royal College of Obstetricians and Gynaecologists,[100] the Royal College of General Practice,[101] the British Association of Accident and Emergency Medicine[102] and the British Medical Association[103] have issued guidelines on the identification and care of victims of domestic violence.

What of the charge that other agencies are better placed to tackle the problem? The facts do not bear this out, with evidence that victims present to a variety of agencies with little overlap between those chosen. In one study, of those who had involved the police, only 22% had ever contacted the health or social services.[104]

It seems clear, then, that domestic violence is a health issue and that health professionals are expected to identify victims and intervene. As well as the questioning targeted at selected women described above, the routine inclusion of a question such as, "How are things at home?" in the social history would not be time-consuming and might lead to the identification of many more abused women. However, practice change that is based purely on identifying victims without adequate follow-up arrangements is not sustainable[24,43,80,95,105,106] and may be harmful.[107] It must be based on an infrastructure that fits the demands on the service,[108] improves outcome without consuming staff time excessively and provides feedback for staff of improvement. It must be backed by an educational programme that changes staff expectations of quick-fix solutions and encourages them to value their role in re-empowering women, whatever choices those women then make. Hadley's work provides a model for this, with a domestic violence liaison team taking over once a victim of domestic violence is identified and also providing feedback to and education within the units it supports.[69]

Confidentiality

The second dilemma is whether and when to break confidentiality. This applies principally to disclosure to the child health services and to the police.

The effect on children who witness violence within the home can be devastating. While many parents think that their child is unaware of the abuse, in fact 85–90% of children in violent homes are in the same or next room when the violence occurs.[109,110] Half of the children present during violence are injured trying to protect their mother.[111] Around 40% of the children of battered women are themselves victims of escalated abuse from their fathers. This child abuse is thought in many instances to be a method of coercing or retaliating against the mother (the Medea complex).[112] The vast majority of children are thought to be adversely affected[113,114] with the ill effect manifesting itself in many ways as the child grows. The child's response to witnessing family violence includes:

- emotional and behavioural problems including:
  - ☐ enuresis
  - ☐ sleep disorders
  - ☐ chronic somatic disorders
  - ☐ truancy and other problems in school
  - ☐ violent and aggressive behaviour
  - ☐ substance abuse
  - ☐ suicide.[115]

There is evidence that mothers who are abused are themselves more likely to abuse their children than those who are not,[116] although the risk to the child is considerably less than the risk posed by the perpetrator of abuse to the mother.[117] In turn, 50–70% of the mothers of abused children are themselves abused.[111,118]

The adverse effect on the child of witnessing or being involved in domestic violence is, therefore, well documented[119,120] and some child health professionals support the routine reporting of the involvement of a parent in domestic violence to the child protection team or, at least, to the child's health visitor. On the other hand, organisations that support women victims of violence, such as Women's Aid, are very much against the disclosure of discussions between a health professional and their patient to any other party without the woman's consent and point out the reluctance to reveal violence which attends a woman's fear that revelation may lead to her children being taken into care.

The health professional must discuss the safety of any children in the home with the domestic violence victim. Where the children have been assaulted themselves and the victim is herself the abuser, or intends returning with her children to the perpetrator, the physician must refer the child to the paediatric service for assessment. Where the victim has not abused the children and wishes to separate from the perpetrator she should be advised to seek legal advice as detailed above. Section 52 and schedule 6 of Part IV of the Family Law Act 1996 amend the Children Act 1989 to enable the court, when making an interim care order or an emergency protection order, to attach an order excluding a suspected abuser from the home. Such an order may have a power of arrest attached.

The risk to the victim of the perpetrator seeing the child's health records must be remembered. Both parents are likely to have the right to examine a child's records and it is unwise to record a history of abuse of the mother in the child's notes while the abusive situation remains unresolved. The child at-risk register is kept in confidence with restricted access and details of the child's situation can be recorded within these files. Most paediatric and emergency services have a system of 'special case' records where a coded marker on the notes alerts the health professional to seek further details in a confidential separate file.

Finally, a suspected victim may well arrive together with her children. The physician is then faced with the dilemma of whether to question the mother in front of the children. The consensus seems to be that general questions should be asked but detailed interview should take place separately from children.[121] The American Academy of Pediatricians has recommended that physicians incorporate domestic violence screening into their child assessment.

The second situation where the physician has to make a decision whether to break confidentiality is in assessing the severity of injury to a domestic violence victim and the degree of risk to a victim who is returning to the perpetrator. Since the introduction of the Police and Criminal Evidence (PACE) Act 1984, the judicial system has accepted that Section 116 and Schedules 5 Parts I and II, containing the definition of 'serious arrestable offence' can be used as a guideline for the release of nonclinical information without the patient's consent. The request should come from a police officer of inspector rank or above and be referred to the patient's consultant for decision. Table 15.1 lists these offences.

It can be seen that, while some criteria such as the use of firearms are clear, some are very much a matter of judgement. In all cases, the physician must seek to come to an agreement with the woman to release information, provided that the woman is physically or mentally fit enough to hold a discussion. It is important to the progress of the victim that she is empowered by being in control of any decisions which are made about her situation but the physician's fears for her safety may outweigh this consideration. The increased risk to the victim of severe injury and death

Table 15.1 Serious arrestable offences; definitions under the Police and Criminal Evidence Act 1984

Seriousness	Section	Offences
Always	Part I	Treason
		Murder
		Manslaughter
		Rape
		Kidnapping
		Incest with a girl under 13 years
		Buggery with a boy under the age of 16 years or a person who has not consented
		Indecent assault which constitutes an act of gross indecency
	Part II	Causing an explosion likely to endanger life or property
		Intercourse with a girl under the age of 13 years
		Possession of firearms with intent to injure
		Use of firearms and imitation firearms to resist arrest
		Carrying firearms with criminal intent
		Hostage taking
		Hijacking
May be	Section 116	Any offence which has lead to:
		Serious harm to the State or public order
		Serious interference with the administration of justice, or with the investigation of offences or of a particular offence
		The death of any person
		Serious injury to any person
		Substantial financial gain to any person
		Serious financial loss to any person
		In this section 'injury' includes any impairment of a person's physical or mental condition

that accompanies separation from the perpetrator must also weigh heavily in the balance.[77] It must be remembered that the release of information applies only to nonclinical information.

References

1. Davies J, Lyon E, Monti-Catania D. Safety *Planning with Battered Women: Complex Lives/Difficult Choices*. Thousand Oaks, CA: Sage publications; 1998.
2. Wilson KJ. *When Violence Begins at Home: A Comprehensive Guide to Understanding and Ending Domestic Abuse*. Alameda, CA: Hunter House; 1997.
3. Dutton DG, Golant SK. *The Batterer: A Psychological Profile*. New York: Basic Books; 1995.
4. Walker LE. *The Battered Woman*. New York: Harper and Row; 1979.
5. Stark E, Flitcraft A, Frazier W. Medicine and patriarchal violence: the social construction of a "private" event. *Int J Health Serv* 1979;9:461–93.
6. Follingstad D, Rutledge C, Berg B. The role of emotional abuse in physically abusive relationships. *J Fam Violence* 1990;5:107–20.

7.   Gortner ET, Gollan JK, Jacobson NS. Psychological aspects of perpetrators of domestic violence and their relationships with the victims. *Psychiatr Clin North Am* 1997;20:337–352.

8.   Barnett DW, LaViolette AD: *It Could Happen to Anyone: Why Battered Women Stay*. Newbury Park, CA: Sage Publications; 1993.

9.   Dutton DG, Painter S. The battered woman syndrome: effects of severity and intermittency of abuse. *Am J Orthopsychiatry* 1993;63:614–22.

10.   Stanko E. *Counting the Costs*. Swindon: Crime Concern; 1998.

11.   Bergman B, Brismar B. A 5-year follow-up study of 117 battered women. *Am J Public Health* 1991;81:1486–9.

12.   Stockwell F. *The Unpopular Patient*. London: Croom Helm; 1984.

13.   Koss MP, Heslet L. Somatic consequences of violence against women. *Arch Fam Med* 1992;1:53–9.

14.   Reece J. Female survivors of abuse attending A and E with self injury. *Accid Emerg Nurs* 1998;6:133–8.

15.   Plichta S. The effects of woman abuse on health care utilisation and health status: a literature review. *Women's Health Issues* 1992;2:154–63.

16.   Bergman B, Brismar B. Battered wives: measures by the social and medical services. *Postgrad Med J* 1990;66:28–33.

17.   Koss MP, Koss PG, Woodruff WJ. Deleterious effects of criminal utilization on women's health and medical utilization. *Arch Intern Med* 1991;151:342–7.

18.   Drossman DA, Leserman J, Nachman G, Li ZM, Gluck H, Toomey TC, *et al.* Sexual and physical abuse in women with functional or organic gastrointestinal disorders. *Ann Intern Med* 1990;113:823–33.

19.   Morrison LJ. The battering syndrome: a poor record of detection in the emergency department. *J Emerg Med* 1988;6:521–6.

20.   Smith PH, Gittelman DK. Psychological consequences of battering: Implications for women's health and medical practice. *N C Med J* 1994;55:434–9.

21.   Domino JV, Haber JD. Prior physical and sexual abuse in women with chronic headache: clinical correlates. *Headache* 1987;27:310–14.

22.   Campbell JC, Lewandowski LA. Mental and physical health effects of intimate partner abuse on women and children. *Psychiatr Clin North Am* 1997;20:353–74.

23.   Drossman DA, McKee DC, Sandler RS, Mitchell CM, Cramer E, Lowman BC, *et al.* Psychosocial factors in the irritable bowel syndrome. A multivariate study of patients and non-patients with irritable bowel syndrome. *Gastroenterology* 1988;95:701–8.

24.   Roberts GL, Lawrence JM, O'Toole BI, Raphael B. Domestic violence in the emergency department: 1. Two case–control studies of victims. *Gen Hosp Psychiatry* 1997;19:5–11.

25.   Campbell J, Kub JE, Rose L. Depression in battered women. *J Am Med Womens Assoc* 1996;51:106–10.

26.   Jaffe P, Wolfe DA, Wilson S, Zak L. Emotional and physical health problems of battered women. *Can J Psychiatry* 1986;31:625–9.

27.   Walker LE. Post-traumatic stress disorder in women: diagnosis and treatment of battered women. *Psychotherapy* 1991;28:21–9.

28.   Carmen EH Rieker PP Mills T. Victims of violence and psychiatric illness. *Am J Psychiatry* 1984;141:378–83.

29.   Ratner PA. The incidence of wife abuse and mental health status in abused wives in Edmonton, Alberta. *Can J Public Health* 1993;84:246–9.

30.   Hathaway JE, Mucci LA, Silverman JG, Brooks DR, Mathews R, Pavlos CA. Health status and health care use of Massachusetts women reporting partner abuse. *Am J Prev Med* 2000;19:302–7.

31.   Bergman B, Brismar B. Suicide attempts by battered wives. *Acta Psychiatr Scand* 1991;83:380–4.

32.   Reichenberg-Ullman J, Ullman R. *Prozac Free*. Rocklin, CA: Prima Publishing; 1999.

33.   Jacobson A. Physical and sexual assault histories among psychiatric outpatients. *Am J Psychiatry* 1989;146:755–8.

34.   Jacobson A, Richardson B. Assault experiences of 100 psychiatric in-patients – evidence of the need for routine enquiry. *Am J Psychiatry* 1987;144:908–13.

35.   Flitcraft A. Clinical violence interventions: lessons from battered women. *J Health Care Poor Underserved* 1995;6:187–97.

36. Mark J, Williams G, Pollock LR. Psychological aspects of the suicidal process. In: van Heeringen K, editor. *Understanding Suicidal Behaviour*. New York: John Wiley; 2001.
37. Jehu D. *Patients as Victims*. Chichester: Wiley; 1994.
38. Romans SE, Anderson JC, Martins JL, Herbison GP, Mullen PE. Sexual abuse in childhood and deliberate self harm. *Am J Psychiatry* 1995;152:1336–42.
39. Muelleman RL, Lenaghan PA, Pakieser RA. Battered women: Injury location and types. *Ann Emerg Med* 1996;28:486–92.
40. Richardson J, Feder G. Domestic violence: a hidden problem for general practice. *Br J Gen Pract* 1996;46:239–42.
41. Fanslow JL, Norton RN, Spinola CG. Indicators of assault-related injuries among women presenting to the emergency department. *Ann Emerg Med* 1998;32:341–8.
42. Spedding RL, McWilliams M, McNicholl BP, Dearden CH. Markers for domestic violence in women. *J Accid Emerg Med* 1999;16:400–2.
43. Warshaw C. Establishing an appropriate response to domestic violence in your practice, institution and community. In: Warshaw C, editor. *Improving the Health Care Response to Domestic Violence: A Manual for Health Care Providers*. San Francisco, CA: Family Violence Prevention Fund; 1998.
44. Goldberg WG, Tomlanovich MC. Domestic violence victims in the Emergency Department. New Findings. *JAMA* 1984;251:3259–3264.
45. Bates L, Redman S, Brown W, Hancock L. Domestic violence experienced by women attending an accident and emergency department. *Aust J Public Health* 1995;19:293–9.
46. Abbott J, Johnson R, Koziol-McLain J, Lowenstein SR. Domestic violence against women. Incidence and prevalence in an emergency department population. *JAMA* 1995;273:1763–7.
47. de Vries Robbe M, March L, Vinen J, Horner D, Roberts G. Prevalence of domestic violence among patients attending a hospital emergency department. *Aust N Z J Public Health* 1996;20:364–8.
48. Roberts GL, O'Toole BI, Raphael B, Lawrence JM, Ashby R. Prevalence study of domestic violence victims in an emergency department. *Ann Emerg Med* 1996;27:741–53.
49. Dearwater SR, Coben JH, Campbell JC, Nah G, Glass N, McLoughlin E, *et al*. Prevalence of intimate partner abuse in women treated at community hospital emergency departments. *JAMA* 1998;280:433–8.
50. Ernst AA, Weiss SJ, Nick TG, Casalletto J, Garza A. Domestic violence in a university emergency department. *South Med J* 2000;93:176–81.
51. Heron SL, Baines PA, Loya D. Domestic violence among inner-city women presenting to the emergency department. *Acad Emerg Med* 1995;2:450.
52. Lo Vecchio F, Bhatia A, Sciallo D. Screening for domestic violence in the emergency department. *Eur J Emerg Med* 1998;5:441–4.
53. Wright J Kariya A. Characteristics of female victims of assault attending a Scottish Accident and Emergency Department. *J Accid Emerg Med* 1997;14:375–8.
54. Watts S. *Evaluation of Health Service Interventions in Response to Domestic Violence Against Women in Camden and Islington*. London: Camden and Islington NHS Health Authority; 2002.
55. Mirlees-Black C. *Domestic Violence: Findings from the British Crime Survey Self-completion Questionnaire, 1996*. Home Office Research, Development and Statistics Directorate Research Findings No. 86. London: Home Office; 1999. [www.homeoffice.gov.uk/rds/pdfs/hors191.pdf] Accessed 15 September 2003.
56. Wilt S, Olson S. Prevalence of domestic violence in the United States. *J Am Med Womens Assoc* 1996;51:77–82.
57. Current trends family and other intimate assaults, Atlanta, 1984. *MMWR Morb Mort Wkly Rep* 1990;39(31):525–9. [www.cdc.gov/mmwr/preview/mmwrhtml/00001707.htm]. Accessed 15 September 2003.
58. Richardson J, Coid J, Petruckevitch A, Chung W, Moorey S, Feder G. Identifying domestic violence: cross sectional study in primary care. *BMJ* 2002;324:274.
59. Stark E. Discharge planning with battered women. *Disch Plann Update* 1994;14:3–7.
60. Campbell JC, Pliska MJ, Taylor W, Sheridan D. Battered women's experiences in the emergency department. *J Emerg Nurs* 1994;20:280–8.

61. Bayatpour M, Wells RD, Holford S. Physical and sexual abuse as predictors of substance abuse and suicide among pregnant teenagers. *J Adolesc Health* 1992;13:128–32.
62. McCoy M. Domestic violence: clues to victimisation. *Ann Emerg Med* 1996;27:764–5.
63. Stanko EA. *Intimate Intrusions. Women's Experience of Male Violence*. London: Routledge and Kegan Paul; 1985.
64. Davies K, Edwards L. Domestic Violence: A challenge to accident and emergency nurses. *Accid Emerg Nurs* 1999;7:26–30.
65. Dobash RP. The nature of antecedents of violent events. *Br J Criminol* 1984;24:2.
66. Gazmararian JA, Lazorick S, Spitz AM, Ballard TJ, Saltzman LE, Marks JS. Prevalence of violence against pregnant women. *JAMA* 1996;275:1915–20.
67. Gielen AC, O'Campo PJ, Faden RR, Kass NE, Xue X. Interpersonal; conflict and physical violence during the childbearing year. *Soc Sci Med* 1994;39:781–7.
68. Grunfeld AF, Ritmiller S, Mackay K, Cowan L, Hotch D. Detecting domestic violence in the emergency department: a nursing triage model. *J Emerg Nurs* 1994;20:271–4.
69. Short LM, Hadley SM, Bates B. Assessing the success of the Womankind program: an integrated model of 24-hour health care response to domestic violence. *Women Health* 2002;35:101–19.
70. Olson L, Anctil C, Fullerton, L, Brillman J, Arbuckle J, Sklar D. Increasing emergency physician recognition of domestic violence. *Ann Emerg Med* 1996;27:741–6.
71. Sassetti MR. Domestic violence. *Prim Care* 1993;20:289–305.
72. Rittmayer J, Roux G.. Relinquishing the need to 'fix it': medical intervention with domestic abuse. *Qual Health Res* 1999;9:166–81.
73. Proschaska JO, DiClemente CC, Norcross JC. In search of how people change: applications to addictive behaviour. *Am Psychol* 1992;47:1102–14.
74. Campbell JC, Sheridan DJ. Emergency nursing interventions with battered women. *J Emerg Nurs* 1989;15:12–17.
75. Chescheir N. Violence against women: response from clinicians. *Ann Emerg Med* 1996;27:766–8.
76. Fullin KJ, Cosgrove A. Empowering physicians to respond to domestic violence. *Wis Med J* 1992;91:280–3.
77. Wilson M, Daly M. Spousal homicide risk and estrangement. *Violence Vict* 1993;8:3–16.
78. Gelles RJ. *Intimate Violence in Families*. 3rd ed. Thousand Oaks, CA: Sage Publications; 1993.
79. Dobash RE, Dobash R. *Violence Against Wives*. New York: Free Press; 1979.
80. Gremillion DH, Kanof E. Overcoming barriers to physician involvement in identifying and referring victims of domestic violence. *Ann Emerg Med* 1996;27:769–73.
81. Frank JB, Rodowski MF. Review of psychological issues in victims of domestic violence seen in emergency settings. *Emerg Med Clin North Am* 1999;17:657–77.
82. Home Office Research and Planning Unit. *Policing Domestic Violence in the 1990s*. Home Office Research Study 139. London: HMSO; 1995.
83. Department of Health. *Domestic Violence: A Resource Manual for Health Care Professionals*. London: DoH; 2000. [www.doh.gov.uk/pdfs/domestic.pdf]. Accessed 15 September 2003.
84. Ramsay J, Richardson J, Carter YH, Davidson LL, Feder G. Should health professionals screen women for domestic violence? *BMJ* 2002;325:314.
85. Cole TB. Is domestic violence screening helpful?. *JAMA* 2000;284:551–3.
86. Ramsay J, Richardson J, Carter Y, Feder G. *Appraisal of Evidence About Screening Women for Domestic Violence*. Report to National Screening Committee October 2001. London: Barts and The London Queen Mary's School of Medicine and Dentistry; 2001. [www.nelh.nhs.uk/screening/adult_pps/domesticviolence.pdf]. Accessed 15 September 2003.
87. Friedman LS, Samet JH, Roberts MS, Hudlin M, Hans P. Inquiry about victimisation experiences. A survey of patient preferences and physician practices. *Arch Intern Med* 1992;152:1186–90.
88. Sugg NK, Inui T. Primary care physicians' response to domestic violence: Opening Pandora's box. *JAMA* 1992;267:3157–60.
89. Love C, Gerbert B, Caspers N, Bronstone A, Perry D, Bird W. Dentists' attitudes and behaviours regarding domestic violence. *J Am Dent Assoc* 2001;132:85–93.
90. Rodriguez MA, Bauer HM, McLoughlin E, Grumbach K. Screening and intervention

for intimate partner abuse: practice and attitudes of primary care physicians. *JAMA* 1999;282:468–74.

91. Waalen J, Goodwin MM, Spitz AM, Petersen R, Saltzman LE. Screening for intimate partner violence by health care providers: barriers and interventions. *Am J Prev Med* 2000;19:230–7.

92. Attala JM, Oetker D, McSweeney M. Partner abuse against female nursing students. *J Psychosoc Nurs Ment Health Serv* 1995;33:17–24.

93. deLahunta EA, Tulsky AA. Personal exposure of faculty and medical students to family violence. *JAMA* 1996;275:1903–6.

94. Dutton MA, Mitchell B, Haywood Y. The Emergency department as a violence prevention centre. *J Am Med Womens Assoc* 1996;51:92–95,117.

95. McLeer SV, Anwar RA, Herman S, Maquiling K. Education is not enough: a systems failure in protecting battered women. *Ann Emerg Med* 1989;18:651–3.

96. Bokunewicz B, Copel LC. Attitudes of emergency nurses before and after a 60 minute educational presentation on partner abuse. *J Emerg Nurs* 1992;18:24–7.

97. Department of Health. *Reforming Emergency Care*. London: DoH; 2001.

98. Stevens KLH. The role of the accident and emergency department. In: Bewley S, Friend JR, Mezey GC, editors. *Violence Against Women*. London: RCOG Press; 1997. p. 168–78.

99. Parker B, McFarlane J, Soeken K, Silva C, Reel S. Testing an intervention to prevent further abuse to pregnant women. *Res Nurs Health* 1999;22:59–66.

100. Recommendations arising from the Study Group on Violence against Women. In: Bewley S, Friend JR, Mezey GC, editors. *Violence Against Women*. London: Royal College of Obstetricians and Gynaecologists; 1997. p. 327–33.

101. Heath I. *Domestic Violence: The General Practitioner's Role*. Royal College of General Practitioners Policy Statement. [www.rcgp.org.uk/rcgp/corporate/position/dom_violence/index.asp]. Accessed 15 September 2003.

102. Stevens KLH. *Domestic Violence: Recognition and Management in Accident and Emergency*. London: British Association of Accident and Emergency Medicine; 1994.

103. British Medical Association. *Domestic Violence: A Health Care Issue?* London: BMA; 1998.

104. Brookoff D, O'Brien KK, Cook CS, Thompson TD, Williams C. Characteristics of participants in domestic violence: assessment at the scene of domestic assault. *JAMA* 1997;277:1369–73.

105. Fanslow JL, Norton RN, Robinson EM. One year follow up of an emergency department protocol for abused women. *Aust N Z J Public Health* 1999;23:418–20.

106. Harwell TS, Casten RJ, Armstrong KA, Dempsey SS, Coons HL, Davis M. Results of a domestic violence training programme offered to the staff of urban community health centers. Evaluation Committee of the Philadelphia Family Violence Working Group. *Am J Prev Med* 1998;15:235–42.

107. Campbell JC. Promise and perils of surveillance in addressing violence against women. *Violence Against Women* 2000;6:705–27.

108. Birnbaum A, Calderon Y, Gennis P, Rao R, Gallagher EJ. Domestic violence: diurnal mismatch between need and availability of services. *Acad Emerg Med* 1996;3:246–51.

109. Groves BM, Zuckerman S, Marans S, Cohen DJ. Silent victims: children who witness violence. *JAMA* 1993;269:262–4.

110. Jaffe PG, Hurley DJ, Wolfe D. Children's observations of violence: I and II. *Can J Psychiatry* 1990;35:466–76.

111. McCloskey LA. The "Medea complex" among men: the instrumental abuse of children to injure wives. *Violence Vict* 2001;16:19–37.

112. Lemmey D, McFarlane J, Willson P, Malecha A. Intimate partner violence. Mothers' perspectives of the effects on their children. *MCN Am J Matern Child Nurs* 2001;26:98–103.

113. Wildin SR, Williamson WD, Wilson GS. Children of battered women: developmental and learning profiles. *Clin Pediatr (Phila)* 1991;30:299–304.

114. Jaffe PG, Wolfe DA, Wilson SK. *Children of Battered Women*. Newbury Park, CA: Sage; 1990.

115. Miller BA, Smyth NJ, Mudar PJ. Mothers' alcohol and other drug problems and their punitiveness towards children. *J Stud Alcohol* 1999;60:632–42.

116. Saunders DG. Child custody decisions in families experiencing woman abuse. *Soc Work* 1994;39:51–9.
117. McKibben L, De Vos E, Newberger EH. Victimization of mothers of abused children: a controlled study. *Pediatrics* 1989;84:531–5.
118. Grych JH, Jouriles EN, Swank PR, McDonald R, Norwood WD. Patterns of adjustment among children of battered women. *J Consult Clin Psychol* 2000;68:84–94.
119. Webb E, Shankleman J, Evans MR, Brooks R. The health of children in refuges for women victims of domestic violence: cross sectional descriptive survey. *BMJ* 2001;323:210–13.
120. Zink T. Should children be in the room when the mother is screened for partner violence? *J Fam Pract* 2000;49:130–6.
121. Erickson MJ, Hill TD, Siegel RM. Barriers to domestic violence screening in the paediatric setting. *Pediatrics* 2001;108:98–102.

Chapter 16

Child sexual abuse

Camille de San Lazaro

Introduction

Sexual abuse in young children is most commonly experienced at the hands of someone they trust, a family member or a person in authority. The experience is likely to be repetitive and when an adult is involved, may involve a prolonged period of 'grooming'. This process is one whereby the child becomes increasingly involved in a relationship, feels cherished and special, or alternatively accepts that escalating sexual contact is the norm. Sexual abuse rarely takes place in a vacuum. Children who are emotionally deprived or neglected are more likely to be targeted. Distorted family relationships, violence, drugs or alcohol abuse in the child's environment are factors that increase susceptibility.

Abused children may be involved in a variety of acts ranging from indecent exposure to contact abuse and anal or vaginal penetration.

Adolescents may be coerced into sexual engagement with older adults, which cause them to disengage from family and peers and which are ultimately emotionally damaging.

Behavioural changes or physical symptoms may be subtle and, in young children, easily attributable to other events which cause emotional instability, such as family breakdown or the birth of a sibling.

Symptoms may include vulvovaginitis, new onset of wetting and soiling, clinginess and sleep disturbance. Many children are symptom-free and the first indication may be a spontaneous remark or the fortuitous discovery of signs of genital trauma. Older girls may present with sexually transmitted disease or pregnancy. Those with psychological distress may display a range of behaviours, including self-harming, absconding and substance abuse.

Children who make graphic statements about sexual acts should always be taken seriously and the matter reported to child protection agencies.

Examining the sexually abused child

Principles

It is critical that this process is carefully planned and conducted by someone with expertise, and that the process is directed at healing. Many children are extremely fearful. It should be remembered that they may have been lied to by their abuser. For example, they may have been told that they would be removed from home or that the examination will hurt.

The environment should be child friendly. Time should be spent in play and the child should be supported by an empathetic adult.[1] The assessment should seek to obtain a full understanding of the child's developmental status, current and past symptomatology and likely need for aftercare.[2]

Anogenital examination should be conducted as part of a full head-to-toe and systems examination. The approach should not be intrusive, and distraction and feedback appropriate to age and cognitive ability should be provided. The child is enabled to feel whole because the physician has taken an interest in other issues affecting the child's life and other aspects of the child's health, through the medium of a full history and examination.

Taking the history

The history should be taken from the best informant, either the parent or a child protection professional (police officer or social worker). If a member of the statutory agencies has not formally interviewed the child, care should be taken to avoid contamination. The history may be taken in another room or area out of earshot of the child. However, there are many occasions when the child is the best informant. A history from the child should be collected through free recall without prompts or direct questions, and with a non-judgemental approach. Asking the child why she has come to see you is the best way to start and this could be followed by a question such as, "Can you tell me about it?". The history collection serves to allow the child to feel a sense of why they are there and a sense of consenting to the process. It is not a forensic interview, which in the UK is conducted by police officers and social workers under rigorous guidelines. In the USA, it is accepted that paediatricians have the best skills in achieving rapport with children and conduct forensic interviews.[3] All such interviews should be recorded with good sound and camera equipment and in the UK there are established Home Office guidelines for this process.[4]

Process of anogenital examination

The child is best examined lying supine on a firm couch, with feet firmly on the bed, knees separated and supported. In this position, firm posterior traction (towards the bed) can be applied, stretching the labia and drawing down the fourchette and hymen to obtain a clear view of the orifice and free

(a)

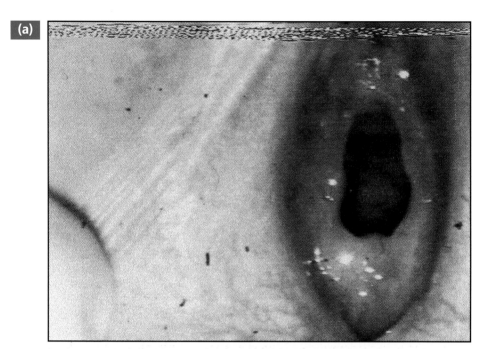

(b)

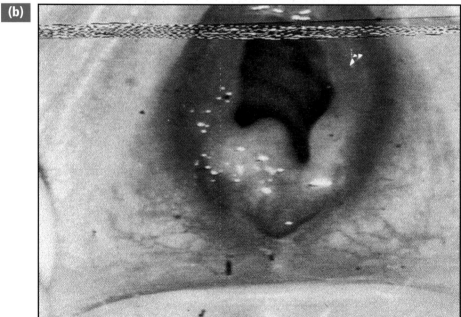

Figure 16.1 Prepubescent hymen examined with (a) posterior traction and (b) anterior traction; the clefts are elicited by stretching the hymen laterally with anterior traction

edge. This procedure is usually sufficient to establish normality. Infants may be less anxious if they are examined on a parent's knee. However, this method is often unsatisfactory, because the persistent oestrogen effect in this age group tends to obscure the orifice and evidence of trauma.

The definition of minor clefts or bumps may be further enhanced by examination in the knee–chest position. Areas of the hymen that have folded over or which are redundant and present as bumps may cause confusion. The knee–chest position tends to resolve these minor changes. Firm anterior traction often achieves this and is usually more acceptable to the child (the labia are grasped and drawn anteriorly towards the pubes) (Figure 16.1a,b).[5]

It is rare that any other manipulation is required but the use of a warm saline rinse to 'float up' the hymen or a damp cotton bud to define the free edge is occasionally necessary.[6]

Anal inspection may be conducted in knee–chest or left lateral position or by simply extending the lithotomy position in younger children. Buttock separation should be gentle to avoid spasm. It should be brief and the time lag before individual signs appear should be noted. Prolonged pressure on the perianal area, for example, may result in venous suffusion at the anus.[7]

All children should be offered privacy and reassurance. The approach should be matter-of-fact and it is important to let the child know how normal she is, using appropriate language. Abnormalities should be similarly reflected using words that are meaningful. "Scar" is a fearsome word; "a little bump which will go away soon" is helpful, accurate and reassuring.

Normal anogenital findings

The hymen in the infant and young toddler usually demonstrates an oestrogen effect. It is abundant and redundant, often with a frilly edge. Congenital absence of the hymen is probably not a clinical entity.[8,9] The labia are plump and the orifice is difficult to visualise without considerable manipulation or gentle probing with a moist cotton bud.

In mid-childhood, the hymen loses the oestrogen effect, the labia are flattened and all structures atrophic. The hymen in this age group usually presents as a delicate, fine structure, with well-defined symmetrical vascularity. The hymenal orifice is annular or, more often, crescentic and the free edge is sharp and well defined. With simple posterior traction, a view of the posterior vaginal wall is normally obtained. The free edge of the orifice may demonstrate shallow notches or small bumps or protrusions; these are most acceptable anteriorly, although a normal bump or notch may occasionally be visible in the posterior free edge. Strong periurethral bands are normal, as are fine adhesions around the insertion of the hymen.[10] The fourchette may be rounded and smooth but most often presents as a sharp clean structure when the perineum is stretched. A pale fine line of avascularity in the midline may be present and mistaken for scarring (linear vestibularis).

The adolescent hymen (see Chapter 6) once more displays the oestrogen effect. It is abundant and numerous folds make the configuration difficult to define. A cotton-tipped swab may be used to demonstrate continuity of the hymenal ring and degree of ability to stretch. A leucorrhoeic discharge is likely to be present. Emans demonstrated that tampon use does not produce significant signs of hymenal trauma.[11]

The most readily definable congenital anomaly is a septate hymen. This anomaly is only rarely associated with more extensive abnormality. Complete occlusion is extremely rare (imperforate hymen). There have been anecdotal reports of complete or almost complete occlusion secondary to healing trauma – the so-called acquired imperforate hymen.[12,13] Fleshy hymenal tags are relatively common.

Genital findings in sexual abuse

"It is normal to be normal".[14] Many sexually abused children, even when graphic accounts of frequent contact and pain are given, will be normal at examination. It is uncertain why this is, but it seems possible that much adult sexual contact with children, although painful, does not involve hymenal tearing. The infliction of acute injury is likely to lead to early detection and it seems likely that perpetrators seek to avoid this.

The structures around the introitus in prepubescence tend to be atrophic and highly sensitive to touch. It is also recognised that tearing and other significant trauma may heal to oblivion[15] and most children make statements some time after the event, often when they feel safe from the abuser.

Substantial changes are not expected with most child sexual abuse. Changes of repetitive abuse include hymenal loss or attenuation. The hymen may appear as a narrowed, rolled nodular strip with poor definition. Such changes are inevitably associated with a gaping, enlarged orifice, presenting as an obvious abnormality not requiring manipulation of the labia. The size of the hymenal orifice is generally a poor indicator of previous trauma. It is highly dependent upon the state of relaxation of the child and the skill of the examiner.[16] A large orifice is often normal in the obese child and should be disregarded if there is good depth of tissue to the posterior hymen.

Healed tears may be visualised as deep V-shaped clefts within the posterior hymen. Complete transections with separation of segments of the hymen are rare and are more likely to be noted after severe penetrative assaults rather than in long-standing sexual abuse. Such transections may be associated with composite scarring through the fourchette, manifested by a mounded, palpable lesion in the midline area.

Hymenal scars present as pale nodular lesions, which distort the hymenal free edge and which may be associated with a change in vascularity. They are rare.

Disruption to the adolescent hymen is often diffuse and difficult to define. Complete transections are unusual, even in the regularly sexually active adolescent. Probing with glaister rods or cotton swabs may be required to demonstrate hiatuses or the degree of accommodation of the hymenal orifice.

It is unwise, with any young person, to make a firm judgement of the likelihood or otherwise of blunt penetration.

Signs are often subtle. They may be masked by spasm and an inability to relax. Significant trauma may heal rapidly. A study of pregnant adolescents showed that only a tiny percentage had definite evidence of any penetration.[17]

Acute sexual assaults

Findings within hours or days of an assault include nonspecific reddening, oedema of the hymen and surrounding tissues, bruising to the labia minora (Figure 16.2), hymen or urethra and fresh lacerations to the hymen or fourchette. Serious indiscriminate or brutal assaults may be associated with vaginal or rectal tears; persistent bleeding or pain should mandate examination under anaesthesia for such injuries. Such injuries may also be the result of the insertion of foreign objects.

Very young children assaulted in this way, especially by a complete stranger, may sustain severe injury and it is wise to examine such children under elective anaesthesia, ensuring that all facilities for trace evidence collection are to hand and taking care to preserve all protective pads and dressings. Swabs for trace evidence should be complete before the cleansing required for the surgical procedure.

Suction bites may be noted over the neck or pubic area. Aggressive bites may also be seen in brutal assaults. Serial skilled photography and the assistance of a forensic odontologist should be sought in these cases.

Bruising, abrasions and lacerations may be present in extragenital sites. Forceful oral penetration may result in petechial haemorrhages and bruising within the mouth and on the palate.

The long process of swab collection (see Chapter 7) can prove intolerable for very young children. Therefore, even though their injuries may be minor, some small children may need anaesthesia if forensic sampling is to be successful and the child spared further emotional trauma. There are obvious ethical issues. Anaesthesia is not without its risks and in many of these cases the process is serving a criminal justice rather than a clinical requirement.

Anal findings

Anal abnormalities in chronic penetrative abuse include loss of anal tone (laxity), healed scars and tags. Reflex anal dilatation, a spontaneous sustained opening up of the external and internal sphincters, is a pheno-menon described in the repetitively abused child.[18] A consistent reproducing of this finding in the presence of a statement or other behavioural concerns should be considered of significance.[19] A degree of anal dilatation may be

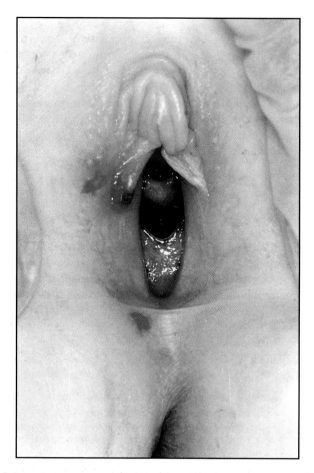

Figure 16.2 Recent stranger assault; petechiae and minor oedema seen in a normal atrophic prepubescent hymen, with crescentic configuration

observed in non-abused children if they are examined at a point where a stool is imminent and present at the internal sphincter. Reflex anal dilatation has been seen in seriously ill children on ventilators, in the haemolytic–uraemic syndrome and is, not unexpectedly perhaps, seen at postmortem examination. It is a phenomenon that may have several explanations. It therefore may not be used as a diagnostic marker for anal abuse unless there are other supportive elements to the diagnosis.

By and large, anal findings are rarely diagnostic of penetration, unlike hymenal tears. However, a scar extending beyond the anal verge should be viewed with suspicion and is unlikely to be the outcome of simple constipation. It should also be recognised that constipation may be a symptom of anal injury.

Acute sodomy may be associated with significant diagnostic signs. Bruising, oedema and lacerations may result. These findings resolve rapidly, often in hours, and the absence of any notable sign does not preclude recent blunt penetration if the examination is delayed by a day or even several hours.

Forensic sampling

The collection of samples should be systematic and based on the history and clinical findings. However, it should be remembered that most small children have little grasp of what has happened and many do not have adequate language. Speculative sampling from extragenital sites such as the inner thighs and umbilicus may be helpful, particularly in young toddlers, where semen or saliva may be discharged over a wide area.

Bites should be swabbed for saliva and salivary material may be available on breasts and clothing. Genital and anal swabs may also yield contraceptive or other lubricant, including saliva, used during the assault.

Seminal material deposited in the mouth degrades rapidly and is unlikely to be available 6–12 hours after the assault.

Nappies, tampons and other clothing should be sought, labelled and sealed under standard guideline procedures.

Urine for toxicology should not be forgotten as drug misuse may be involved.

Differential diagnosis of anogenital symptoms

Nonspecific vulvovaginitis is one of the most common recurrent problems in young girls presenting to general practitioners. These symptoms, which are often difficult to manage, are most likely related to the loss of oestrogen effect and symptoms simulating menopausal vulvitis: dryness, itching, erythema and a sticky discharge. Swabs are usually negative and candidiasis rarely proven, despite the ubiquitous use of antifungal agents. Contact sensitivity to detergents may also cause recurrent symptoms. Careful avoidance of bubble baths and the use of oily substitutes and emollient creams are usually supportive. A history of blood staining should raise suspicion of a foreign body.

Lichen sclerosus et atrophicus is a rare disorder in childhood but can cause confusion. The presence of atrophic skin changes, pallor and haemorrhaging leads to the diagnosis. It is important to note that lichen sclerosus et atrophicus can coexist with sexual abuse and that hymenal abnormality is not a feature of the condition.[20] Symptoms of perineal soreness and itching may be related to skin problems, such as eczema or psoriasis and threadworm infestation.

Sexually transmitted disease

In any child, the isolation of recognised organisms such as *Neisseria gonorrhoea*, *Chlamydia trachomatis* or *Trichomonas vaginalis* should raise the strongest suspicion of abusive contact. While neonatal colonisation is recognised, the presence of such organisms in the genital tract should lead to an investigation into the possibility of sexual transfer. The significance of genital herpes simplex and human papillomavirus is not well established. However, it is entirely appropriate to refer these cases for a wider enquiry. Vertical transmission of human papillomavirus is a likely source of infection in the young child and delayed manifestation is known.

Multidisciplinary working

Investigation and management of child abuse is structured under guidelines laid down by the Department of Health and a legal framework established by the Children Act 1989.[21,22] Paediatricians and other health professionals should seek to work closely with other agencies, notably social services and the police. These agencies have statutory responsibilities for child protection. In most districts each agency has special designated teams working in this field.

Medical practitioners should feel able to share concerns with professionals within other agencies. Often, early sharing of information may lay a matter to rest. Colleagues in other agencies may be able to reassure a doctor that his decision to do nothing is appropriate. A child's abnormal behaviour and statements may be placed in immediate context if that concern, having been shared, leads the police to discover that a known offender has moved into the household. All NHS trusts should have a named doctor available to offer advice on child protection matters; often the named person is willing to take on the tasks of liaison with other agencies. All practitioners who offer medical care to children should, however, recognise that they have a duty to act in the child's best interests at all times.

Recording

A meticulous record of the history and findings is best made using purpose-designed documentation. Photography of injuries can be achieved using any high-resolution camera. The colposcope provides a good light source and may be used both to examine and to record findings. Photographic recording of genital findings is considered good practice. It serves as a useful way of obtaining a clinical review of findings without the need for further examination. Appropriate consent must be obtained and secure arrangements for storage established.

Aftercare

Practitioners dealing with child sexual abuse need to ensure that the emotional needs of the child and family are met. Referral to appropriate counselling services is important. Consideration should be given in every case to the possibility of sexually transmitted infection, which, in young children, may be of forensic significance.

Summary

Abnormal physical findings are uncommon in child sexual abuse. Early examination after the event yields the most abnormality. The examiner should be empathetic, gentle and unhurried. The assessment should include a careful determination of the child's developmental and emotional status. Meticulous recording of findings should include photography with consent.

The examiner has a responsibility to ensure that the further needs of the child are properly met.

References

1. De San Lazaro C. Making paediatric assessment in suspected sexual abuse a therapeutic experience. *Arch Dis Child* 1995;73:174–6.
2. Royal College of Paediatrics and Child Health, Association of Police Surgeons. *Guidance on Paediatric Forensic Examinations in Relation to Possible Child Sexual Abuse.* London; 2002.
3. Levitt CJ. The medical interview. In: Heger AM, Emans SJ, editors. *Evaluation of the Sexually Abused Child.* 2nd ed. Oxford: Oxford University Press; 2000. Chapter 4.
4. Home Office, Department of Health. *Memorandum of good practice on video-recorded interviews with child witnesses for criminal proceedings.* London: HMSO; 1992.
5. McCann J, Voris J, Simon M, Wells R. Comparison of genital examination techniques in prepubertal girls. *Pediatrics* 1990;85:222–3.
6. Myhre AH, Berntzen K, Bratlid D. Genital anatomy in non-abused pre-school girls. *Acta Paediatr* 2003;92:1453–62.
7. Bruni M. Anal findings in sexual abuse of children (a descriptive study). *J Forensic Sci* 2003;48:1343–6.
8. Berenson A, Heger A, Andrews S. Appearance of the hymen in newborns. *Pediatrics* 1991;87:458–65.
9. Jenny C, Kuhns M, Arakawa F. Hymens in newborn female infants, *Pediatrics* 1987;80:399–400.
10. Berenson A, Heger A, Hayes J, Bailey R, Emans SJ. Appearance of the hymen in prepubertal girls. *Pediatrics* 1992;89:387–94.
11. Emans SJ, Woods ER, Allred EN, Grace E. Hymenal findings in adolescent women: impact of tampon use and consensual sexual activity. *J Pediatr* 1994;125:153–60.
12. Botash A, Jean-Louis F. Imperforate hymen: congenital or acquired from sexual abuse? *Pediatrics* 2001;108:E53.
13. Berkovitz CD, Elvik SL, Logan MA. Simulated acquired imperforate hymen following the genital trauma of sexual abuse. *Clin Pediatr* 1987;26:307–9.
14. Adams J, Harper K, Knudson S, Revilla J. Examination findings in legally confirmed sexual abuse: it's normal to be normal. *Pediatrics* 1994;94:310–17.
15. McCann J, Voris J, Simon M. Genital injuries resulting from sexual abuse: a longitudinal study. *Pediatrics* 1992;89:307–17.
16. Heger A, Emans S. Introital diameter as the criterion for sexual abuse. *Pediatrics* 1992;89:307–17.
17. Kellog ND, Shirley W, Menard RN. Genital anatomy in pregnant adolescents: 'normal'

does not mean 'nothing happened'. *Pediatrics* 2004;113:67–9.

18. Hobbs C, Wynne JM. Sexual abuse of English boys and girls: the importance of anal examination. *Child Abuse Negl* 1989;13:195–210.

19. Royal College of Physicians of London. *Physical Signs of Sexual Abuse in Children.* 2nd ed. London: RCP; 1997.

20. Warrington S, San Lazaro C. Lichen sclerosus et atrophicus and sexual abuse. *Arch Dis Child* 1996;75:512–16.

21. Department of Health, Home Office, Department for Education and Employment. *Working Together to Safeguard Children.* London: The Stationery Office; 1999. [www.asylumsupport.info/publications/doh/safeguard.htm].

22. Department of Health, Home Office, Department for Education and Skills. Keeping Children Safe. CM5861. The Government's Response to the Victoria Climbie Inquiry Report and Joint Chief Inspector's Report Safeguarding Children. London: The Stationery Office; 2003 [www.dfes.gov.uk/everychildmatters/downloads.cfm].

Further reading

Books

Adler Z. *Rape on Trial*. London: Routledge & Kegan Paul; 1987. ISBN 0-7102-0804-9

Crowley SA. *Sexual Assault: The Medical Legal Examination*. Appleton & Lange; 1999. ISBN 0-8385-8533-7.

Giardino AP, Datner E, Asher J. *Sexual Assault: Victimisation Across the Lifespan*. GW Medical Publishing; 2000. ISBN 1878060414.

Girardin BW, Faugno, DK, Seneski PC, Slaughter L, Whelan M. *Color Atlas of Sexual Assault*. St. Louis, MO: Mosby; 1997. ISBN 0-8151-3842-3

Hazelwood RR, Burgess AW. *Practical Aspects of Rape Investigation*. Boca Raton: CRC; 1995. ISBN 0-8493-8152-5

HM Crown Prosecution Service Inspectorate. *A Report on the Joint Investigation into the Investigation and Prosecution of Cases Involving Allegations of Rape*. London: HMCPS; 2002.

Harris J, Grace S. *A Question of Evidence? Investigating and Prosecuting Rape in the 1990s*. Home Office Research Study 196. London: Home Office; 1999.

Home Office. *Setting the Boundaries*. London: Home Office Communications Directorate; July 2000.

Kelly L. *A Research Review on the Reporting, Investigation and Prosecution of Rape Cases*. London: HMCPSI; 2002.

LeBeau M, Mozayani A. *Drug-facilitated Sexual Assault*. San Diego, CA: Academic Press; 2001. ISBN 0-12-440261-5

Lees S. *Carnal Knowledge*. London: Penguin; 1997. ISBN 0-140023915-4

McLay WDS. *Clinical Forensic Medicine*. London: Greenwich Medical Media; 1996. ISBN 1-900151-200

Metropolitan Police Authority. *Scrutiny Report: Rape Investigation and Victim Care*. London: Metropolitan Police Authority; April 2002.

Mezey GC, King M. *Male Victims of Sexual Assault*. Oxford: Oxford University Press; 2000. ISBN 0-19-262932-8

Nuttall M. *It Could Have Been You*. London: Virago; 1997. ISBN 1-86049-368-8

Payne-James J, Busuttil A, Smock W. *Forensic Medicine: Clinical and Pathological Aspects*. London: Greenwich Medical Media; 2003. ISBN 1-841100-26-9

Petrak J, Hedge B. *The Trauma of Sexual Assault*. Chichester: John Wiley & Sons; 2002. ISBN 0-471-62691-0

Saward J, Green W. *Rape, My Story*. London: Pan Macmillan; 1995. ISBN 0330341561

Solomon RC, Murphy MC. *What is Justice? Classic and Contemporary Readings*. 2nd ed. Oxford: Oxford University Press; 1999. ISBN 0-19-512810-9

Stark M. *A Physician's Guide to Clinical Forensic Medicine*. New Jersey: Humana Press; 2000. ISBN 0-89603-742-8

Stevenson K, Davies A, Gunn M. *Blackstone's Guide to the Sexual Offences Act 2003*. Oxford: Oxford University Press; 2004. ISBN 0-19-927000

Journals

Child Abuse and Neglect
Official publication of the International Society for the Prevention of Child Abuse and Neglect. Published by Pergamon; ISSN: 0145-2134
[www.elsevier.com/wps/find/journaldescription.cws_home/586/description description]

Child Abuse Review
Published by John Wiley & Sons; ISSN 0952-9136
[www3.interscience.wiley.com/cgi-bin/jhome/5060].

Journal of Clinical Forensic Medicine
Official journal of the Association of Forensic Physicians (formerly the

Association of Police Surgeons), the Australia and New Zealand Forensic Medicine Society Inc. and the British Association in Forensic Medicine. ISSN 1353-1131 [www.harcourt-international.com/journals/jcfm/].

Journal of Forensic Science
The official publication of the American Academy of Forensic Sciences. Published by American Society for Testing and Materials (ASTM); ISSN 0022-1198

Journal of Pediatric and Adolescent Gynecology
Published by Lippincott, Williams & Williams; ISSN 1083-3188

Medicine, Science and the Law: the Official Journal of the British Academy of Forensic Sciences.
Published by Kluwer; ISSN: 0025-8024

Useful organisations and websites

Association of Forensic Physicians: www.afpweb.org.uk

International Society for the Prevention of Child Abuse and Neglect: http://ispcan.org/

Project Sapphire: www.met.police.uk/sapphire

Rape Crisis: www.rapecrisis.co.uk/

Rape, Examination, Counselling and Help (REACH): www.reachcentre.org.uk/

Victim Support: www.victimsupport.org

Women's Aid: www.womensaid.org.uk

Index